Medical and Surgical Management of Common Fertility Issues

Editor

G. WRIGHT BATES Jr

OBSTETRICS AND GYNECOLOGY CLINICS OF NORTH AMERICA

www.obgyn.theclinics.com

Consulting Editor
WILLIAM F. RAYBURN

December 2012 • Volume 39 • Number 4

ELSEVIER

Elsevier, Inc. • 1600 John F. Kennedy Blvd. • Suite 1800 • Philadelphia, PA 19103-2899

http://www.theclinics.com

OBSTETRICS AND GYNECOLOGY CLINICS OF NORTH AMERICA Volume 39, Number 4
December 2012 ISSN 0889-8545, ISBN-13: 978-1-4557-4901-0

Editor: Stephanie Donley

Obstetrics and Gynecology Clinics (ISSN 0889-8545) is published quarterly by Elsevier Inc., 360 Park Avenue South, New York, NY 10010-1710. Months of issue are March, June, September, and December. Periodicals postage paid at New York, NY, and additional mailing offices. Subscription price per year is $275.00 (US individuals), $474.00 (US institutions), $137.00 (US students), $331.00 (Canadian individuals), $598.00 (Canadian institutions), $201.00 (Canadian students), $402.00 (foreign individuals), $598.00 (foreign institutions), and $201.00 (foreign students). To receive student/resident rate, orders must be accompanied by name of affiliated institution, date of term, and the signature of program/residency coordinator on institution letterhead. Orders will be billed at individual rate until proof of status is received. Foreign air speed delivery is included in all *Clinics* subscription prices. All prices are subject to change without notice. POSTMASTER: Send address changes to *Obstetrics and Gynecology Clinics*, Elsevier Health Sciences Division, Subscription Customer Service, 3251 Riverport Lane, Maryland Heights, MO 63043. **Customer Service: Telephone: 1-800-654-2452 (U.S. and Canada); 314-447-8871 (outside U.S. and Canada). Fax: 314-447-8029. E-mail: journalscustomerservice-usa@elsevier.com (for print support); journalsonlinesupport-usa@elsevier.com (for online support).**

Reprints. For copies of 100 or more of articles in this publication, please contact the Commercial Reprints Department, Elsevier Inc., 360 Park Avenue South, New York, New York 10010-1710. Tel.: 212-633-3818; Fax: 212-462-1935; E-mail: reprints@elsevier.com.

Obstetrics and Gynecology Clinics of North America is also published in Spanish by McGraw-Hill Interamericana Editores S.A., P.O. Box 5-237, 06500, Mexico; in Portuguese by Reichmann and Affonso Editores, Rio de Janeiro, Brazil; and in Greek by Paschalidis Medical Publications, Athens, Greece.

Obstetrics and Gynecology Clinics of North America is covered in MEDLINE/PubMed (Index Medicus), Excerpta Medica, Current Concepts/Clinical Medicine, Science Citation Index, BIOSIS, CINAHL, and ISI/BIOMED.

Printed and bound by CPI Group (UK) Ltd, Croydon, CR0 4YY

Transferred to digital print 2012

Contributors

CONSULTING EDITOR

WILLIAM F. RAYBURN, MD, MBA
Randolph Seligman Professor and Chair, Department of Obstetrics and Gynecology, University of New Mexico School of Medicine, Albuquerque, New Mexico

GUEST EDITOR

G. WRIGHT BATES Jr, MD
Associate Professor, Division and Fellowship Director, Reproductive Endocrinology and Infertility, Department of Obstetrics and Gynecology, University of Alabama at Birmingham, Birmingham, Alabama

AUTHORS

G. WRIGHT BATES Jr, MD
Associate Professor, Division and Fellowship Director, Reproductive Endocrinology and Infertility, Department of Obstetrics and Gynecology, University of Alabama School of Medicine, Birmingham, Alabama

KENNETH R. CARSON, MD
Division of Hematology and Oncology, Department of Internal Medicine; Division of Public Health Sciences, Department of Surgery, Washington University in St. Louis, St Louis, Missouri

XIAOXIAO CATHERINE GUO, BS
Program in Reproductive and Adult Endocrinology, Eunice Kennedy Shriver National Institute of Child Health and Human Development, National Institutes of Health, Bethesda, Maryland

ERICA C. DUN, MD, MPH
Fellow, Atlanta Center for Minimally Invasive Surgery and Reproductive Medicine, Atlanta, Georgia

EMILY S. JUNGHEIM, MD, MSCI
Division of Reproductive Endocrinology and Infertility, Department of Obstetrics and Gynecology, Washington University in St. Louis, St Louis, Missouri

MATTHEW LATHAM MACER, MD
Resident, Department of Obstetrics, Gynecology and Reproductive Sciences, Yale School of Medicine, New Haven, Connecticut

JANET F. MCLAREN, MD
Assistant Professor, Division of Reproductive Endocrinology and Infertility, Department of Obstetrics and Gynecology, University of Alabama at Birmingham, Birmingham, Alabama

MAMIE MCLEAN, MD
Division of Reproductive Endocrinology and Infertility, Department of Obstetrics and Gynecology, University of Alabama at Birmingham, Birmingham, Alabama

KELLE H. MOLEY, MD
Division of Reproductive Endocrinology and Infertility, Department of Obstetrics and Gynecology, Washington University in St. Louis, St Louis, Missouri

LAWRENCE M. NELSON, MD, FACOG
Captain, United States Public Health Service, Intramural Research Program on Reproductive and Adult Endocrinology, Eunice Kennedy Shriver National Institute of Child Health and Human Development, National Institutes of Health, Bethesda, Maryland

CEANA H. NEZHAT, MD
Atlanta Center for Minimally Invasive Surgery and Reproductive Medicine; Clinical Associate Professor of Obstetrics and Gynecology, Emory University, Atlanta, Georgia; and Clinical Associate Professor of Obstetrics and Gynecology, Stanford University, California

ANTHONY M. PROPST, MD
Associate Professor, Division of Reproductive Endocrinology and Infertility; Vice Chair, Department of Obstetrics and Gynecology, Uniformed Services University of the Health Sciences, Bethesda, Maryland

SAIMA RAFIQUE, MBBS, DGO
Associate Protocol Coordinator, Intramural Research Program on Reproductive and Adult Endocrinology, Eunice Kennedy Shriver National Institute of Child Health and Human Development, National Institutes of Health, Bethesda, Maryland

JAMES H. SEGARS, MD
Program in Reproductive and Adult Endocrinology, Eunice Kennedy Shriver National Institute of Child Health and Human Development, National Institutes of Health, Bethesda, Maryland

EVELINA W. STERLING, PhD
Associate Investigator, Intramural Research Program on Reproductive and Adult Endocrinology, Eunice Kennedy Shriver National Institute of Child Health and Human Development, National Institutes of Health, Bethesda, Maryland; President, Rachel's Well, McLean, Virginia

HUGH S. TAYLOR, MD
Professor and Chair, Department of Obstetrics, Gynecology and Reproductive Sciences, Yale School of Medicine, New Haven, Connecticut

JENNIFER L. TRAVIESO, BS
Division of Reproductive Endocrinology and Infertility, Department of Obstetrics and Gynecology, Washington University in St. Louis, St Louis, Missouri

MELISSA F. WELLONS, MD
Division of Medical Endocrinology, Department of Internal Medicine, Vanderbilt University, Nashville, Tennessee

Contents

Infertility is a common condition, affecting 15% of couples trying to conceive. The infertility evaluation includes an assessment of both the female and the male partner to discern the factors contributing to their difficulty in conceiving. The basic evaluation includes a careful history of both partners, physical examination of the female partner, investigation of ovulatory function and tubal status, and semen analysis. A more detailed investigation is performed as dictated by individual factors.

Preconception counseling provides an opportunity for health care providers to promote maternal and neonatal health, and to make recommendations regarding the optimization of natural fertility. While educating patients on the negative impact of maternal obesity on fertility and maternal and neonatal health; many health care providers recommend weight loss to reduce these negative outcomes. The recommendations start with lifestyle modifications, including diet and exercise. This article focuses on the available evidence regarding lifestyle modifications and fertility, and on the type of lifestyle modifications that health care providers should recommend to patients seeking to optimize their natural fertility.

Obesity is associated with multiple adverse reproductive outcomes, but the mechanisms involved are largely unknown. Obesity has been referred to as a "complex system," defined as a system of heterogeneous parts interacting in nonlinear ways to influence the behavior of the parts as a whole. Human reproduction is also a complex system; hence the difficulty in identifying the mechanisms linking obesity and adverse reproductive function. This review discusses the adverse reproductive outcomes associated with obesity and the mechanisms involved and concludes with a discussion of public health policy with respect to the treatment of infertility in obese women.

Polycystic ovarian syndrome (PCOS) is a disorder of androgen excess and ovarian dysfunction. Hirsutism and elevated free testosterone levels are the most consistent signs of the androgen excess. Irregular, infrequent, or absent menses and infertility are symptoms of ovulatory dysfunction. Obesity is also a feature of this syndrome and contributes to associated metabolic abnormalities. Lifestyle modification should be the first treatment and is effective in reducing the signs and symptoms. The ovulatory infertility associated with PCOS can be overcome in most cases with oral (clomiphene citrate or letrozole) or injectable (gonadotropins) agents. Surgical intervention is reserved for cases resistant to medical management.

Anovulatory disorders are a primary cause of female infertility. Polycystic ovarian syndrome is the major cause of anovulation and is generally associated with obesity. Lifestyle changes to encourage weight loss are the initial therapy for overweight and obese patients, followed by clomiphene citrate for ovulation induction. For those patients who fail to ovulate on clomiphene citrate, alternatives, such as letrozole; gonadotropins; and complimentary agents to enhance clomiphene citrate, such as metformin and glucocorticoids, are reviewed. Women with unexplained infertility (no identifiable cause of infertility on a routine evaluation) may benefit from ovulation induction with clomiphene citrate, letrozole, or gonadotropins.

Fibroids affect 35% to 77% of reproductive-age women. When selecting a treatment plan for symptomatic fibroids, the fibroid location, size, and number must be considered. Myomectomy remains the preferred method for women with fibroid-related infertility who wish to have children or maintain fertility. Currently available medical therapies reduce symptoms in the short term but may involve side effects when used long term. Initial fertility studies are encouraging but trials are needed. Recent medical advances have led to minimally invasive approaches for women with fibroid disease, but there is a strong demand for additional treatment options.

Endometriois has been associated with infertility; however, the mechanisms by which it affects fertility are still not fully understood. This article reviews the proposed mechanisms of endometriosis pathogenesis, its effects on fertility, and treatments of endometriosis-associated infertility. Theories on the cause of the disease include retrograde menstruation, coelomic metaplasia, altered immunity, stem cells, and genetics. Endometriosis affects gametes and embryos, the fallopian tubes and embryo transport, and the eutopic endometrium; these abnormalities likely all impact fertility. Current treatment options of endometriosis-associated infertility include surgery, superovulation with intrauterine insemination, and in vitro fertilization. We also discuss potential future treatments for endometriosis-related infertility.

Tubal factor infertility accounts for a large portion of female factor infertility. The most prevalent cause of tubal factor infertility is pelvic inflammatory disease and acute salpingitis. The diagnosis of tubal occlusion can be established by a combination of clinical suspicion based on patient history and diagnostic tests, such as hysterosalpingogram, sonohysterosalpingography, and laparoscopy with chromopertubation. Depending on several patient factors, tubal microsurgery or more commonly in vitro fertilization with its improving success rates are the recommended treatment options.

There is a need for a new approach to managing women with primary ovarian insufficiency. This condition is a serious chronic disease that may have far reaching effects on physical and emotional health. An integrative and collaborative approach to management works best. To maintain wellness, most women with primary ovarian insufficiency need to reassess their primary source of meaning and purpose in life and how this diagnosis may have threatened that part of who they are. They also need assessment with regard to bone health, thyroid and adrenal function, determination of *FMR1* premutation and karyotype status, and ongoing estradiol-progestin hormone replacement.

OBSTETRICS AND GYNECOLOGY CLINICS

Foreword

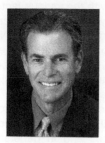

William F. Rayburn, MD, MBA
Consulting Editor

This issue of *Obstetrics and Gynecology Clinics of North America*, guest edited by G. Wright Bates, MD, provides a very contemporary update on the medical and surgical management of common fertility issues. Approximately 15% of couples are unable to achieve pregnancy within 1 year of regular, unprotected intercourse. Any increase in the number of couples seeking evaluation and treatment is associated with delayed childbearing due to a greater emphasis on higher education and career promotion among women. At the same time, fertility declines with advancing age, in part because certain diseases (eg, leiomyomata and endometriosis) that adversely affect fertility also increase with age. In addition, societal acceptances of single parenthood and legal abortion have greatly reduced the number of infants available for adoption.

The authors highlight the complexity of human reproduction. Formal evaluation of infertility is designed to isolate each component of the reproductive process and to identify any abnormalities that may interfere with conception and early pregnancy. Female factors that explain or contribute appreciably to infertility are present in at least half of the couples. A mature ovum must be expelled from the ovaries, ideally on a regular, predictable, cyclic basis. Ovulatory dysfunction, including chronic anovulation, accounts for 40% of infertility in women. Fallopian tubes have dual functions in facilitating ovum capture from the adjacent ovary and in transporting the fertilized egg to the uterine cavity in a timely manner. Peritoneal pathologic conditions and tubal occlusion are among the most common causes of infertility, being responsible in about one-third of infertile couples. The uterus must be receptive to embryo implantation and capable of supporting subsequent normal growth and development. Abnormalities of uterine contour or receptivity may explain or contribute to infertility or early pregnancy loss in up to 10% of couples.

Evaluation of the infertile couple, as described in this issue, should be directed toward identifying the cause and relevant contributors in a systematic, and preferably expeditious and cost-effective manner. The initial emphasis is focused on the least invasive methods to screen for the most common reasons for fertility impairment. The sequence, pace, and extent of evaluation should take into account the couple's

Obstet Gynecol Clin N Am 39 (2012) xi–xii
http://dx.doi.org/10.1016/j.ogc.2012.10.004
0889-8545/12/$ – see front matter © 2012 Published by Elsevier Inc.

wishes, patient's age, duration of infertility, and unique features of their medical histories and physical evaluations that suggest causes for the infertility.

Contemporary approaches to the management of women with the various factors impairing fertility are well-described in each article. I especially enjoyed the descriptions of lifestyle modifications and about obesity and reproductive function. New management approaches to primary ovarian insufficiency, tubal factors, endometriosis, uterine fibroids, and polycystic ovarian syndrome are covered. A treatise about modern assisted reproductive technologies is important for many reasons, especially due to the public's increased awareness and need for open debate.

I wish to thank Dr Bates and his distinguished group of authors for their fine efforts in contributing to this valuable issue. I hope that the practical information provided herein will aid in the implementation of evaluative processes and in generating evidence-based treatment protocols for those women seeking assistance from their obstetrician-gynecologist.

William F. Rayburn, MD, MBA
Department of Obstetrics and Gynecology
University of New Mexico School of Medicine
MSC10 5580; 1 University of New Mexico
Albuquerque, NM 87131-0001, USA

E-mail address:
wrayburn@salud.unm.edu

Preface

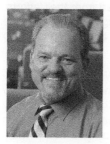

G. Wright Bates Jr, MD
Guest Editor

The classic novel by Leo Tolstoy from the 19th century, *Family Happiness*, is a somewhat ironic portrayal of love, marriage, and family. The main character comments, "children perhaps—what can more the heart of man desire?" This sentiment appears timeless and seems to apply to both genders. This quote from Tolstoy remains true today and was recently used verbatim in an award-winning film, Into the Wild, about self-realization and reflecting on a full life that includes family. Although the desire to produce offspring may not be universal, parenting is highly regarded in most traditions. However, many couples have difficulty achieving a healthy pregnancy and cultural pressures to achieve fertility are an added burden for those who suffer with infertility. Women's health care providers should remain cognizant of the full impact of reproductive dysfunction on many aspects of an individual and/or couple's life, including relationships, ethics, faith, and finances. These couples may also feel alone and unique in their suffering. However, infertility is a common condition and modern treatments for infertility greatly increase the chances of becoming a parent.

In this issue of *Obstetrics and Gynecology Clinics of North America,* experts in the field of women's health care highlight several of the common etiologies of infertility and an evidence-based approach to their treatment. A problem-focused but comprehensive evaluation and team approach are warranted for most patients dealing with infertility. However, it is equally important to avoid unnecessary tests and treatments that lack documented efficacy in helping couples achieve the ultimate goal of a healthy child. Lifestyle modifications and basic treatment, including medical management, will be successful in many instances, while others may require surgical intervention or assisted reproductive technologies. In the end, this edition provides management strategies and a message of hope for success to patients and providers alike.

Obstet Gynecol Clin N Am 39 (2012) xiii–xiv
http://dx.doi.org/10.1016/j.ogc.2012.10.003
0889-8545/12/$ – see front matter © 2012 Elsevier Inc. All rights reserved.

obgyn.theclinics.com

I am grateful to my friends and colleagues, who contributed their time and expertise to this edition. Their commitment to quality patient care and advancement of the science of reproduction is exemplary. Many families have resulted from their efforts. My own mother sought treatment for infertility almost 50 years ago. Her persistence and the compassionate care she received resulted in my birth and inspired me to help others experience the joys of parenthood.

G. Wright Bates Jr, MD
Division of Reproductive Endocrinology and Infertility
Department of Obstetrics and Gynecology
University of Alabama at Birmingham
Birmingham, AL 35249, USA

E-mail address:
wbates@uab.edu

Infertility Evaluation

Janet F. McLaren, MD

KEYWORDS

- Infertility • Fecundity • Ovarian reserve • Hysterosalpingogram • Semen analysis

KEY POINTS

- Infertility is defined as the failure to conceive after 12 months of regular unprotected intercourse.
- Female fecundity is strongly influenced by age, and an infertility evaluation is warranted in women older than 35 years who have not conceived in 6 months.
- An immediate infertility evaluation is warranted in women who are older than 40 years, have evidence of an ovulatory disorder, or are at high risk of pelvic adhesive disease.
- Male factor contributes in more than 50% of infertile couples, thus early evaluation of the male partner will help expedite the identification of all contributing factors.

INTRODUCTION TO INFERTILITY EVALUATION

Infertility is defined as the inability of a couple to conceive after 1 year of regular, unprotected intercourse. Natural cycle fecundity, or the chance of a couple conceiving in a given month, is 20% to 25% for a healthy couple. Approximately 10% to 15% of couples experience infertility, and after 1 year of trying to conceive it is appropriate to evaluate a couple for infertility. Given the known decline of female fecundity with age, it is advised that women 35 years or older be evaluated after 6 months of attempted conception and women 40 years or older undergo an immediate evaluation.

The potential causes for infertility are varied and include endocrine, anatomic, genetic, and behavioral conditions (**Boxes 1–3**). Focusing first on the female partner, ovulatory disorders, anatomic disease of the pelvic organs, and poor oocyte quality can each result in infertility. With regard to the male partner, abnormal sperm quantity or function will affect a couples' fertility potential. An infertility evaluation must cover the breadth of these potential reproductive issues, while maintaining support and empathy for the couple as they struggle with their condition. The following sections outline a focused and evidence-based infertility evaluation.

Disclosures: None.
Division of Reproductive Endocrinology and Infertility, Department of Obstetrics and Gynecology, University of Alabama at Birmingham, 619 19th Street South, Room 10390, Birmingham, AL 35249-7333, USA
E-mail address: jmclaren@uab.edu

Obstet Gynecol Clin N Am 39 (2012) 453–463
http://dx.doi.org/10.1016/j.ogc.2012.09.001
0889-8545/12/$ – see front matter © 2012 Elsevier Inc. All rights reserved.

Box 1
Causes of infertility related to the female partner

- Ovulatory disorders
  - Polycystic ovary syndrome (PCOS)
  - Hyperprolactinemia
  - Hypothalamic hypogonadism
  - Premature ovarian insufficiency (idiopathic or secondary to gonadal dysgenesis)
  - Hypothyroidism
  - Congenital adrenal hyperplasia
- Fallopian tubal disease
  - Proximal or distal tubal obstruction
  - Pelvic adhesive disease
- Uterine causes
  - Fibroids
  - Endometrial polyps
  - Müllerian anomalies
  - Cervical stenosis
  - Intrauterine adhesions
- Oocyte quality
  - Age-related aneuploidy

Box 2
Causes of infertility related to the male partner

- Obstructive disease
  - Vasectomy
  - Congenital absence of the vas deferens
  - Ejaculatory duct obstruction
- Nonobstructive disease
  - Kallmann syndrome or other hypogonadotropic hypogonadism
  - Testicular failure (idiopathic or secondary to gonadal dysgenesis)
  - Hyperprolactinemia
  - Exogenous testosterone exposure
- Functional disorders
  - Erectile dysfunction

Box 3
Causes of infertility related to either or both partners

- "Unexplained" infertility
  - Fertilization defect
- Balanced translocation
- Infrequent coitus

EVALUATION OF THE FEMALE PARTNER
Infertility History

The initial evaluation of the female partner should start with a careful medical history. This history should include the following:

- Duration of infertility
  - How long has the couple been trying?
  - What is the frequency of intercourse, and has intercourse been timed to ovulation?
- Obstetric history
  - Has the patient been pregnant previously, and what was the outcome of that pregnancy?
- Gynecologic history
  - Was pubertal development normal?
  - What is the length of the menstrual cycle, and is this time interval regular?
  - Are menses long in duration, especially heavy or painful?
  - Is there any past history of pelvic infections or pelvic surgery?
  - Does the patient have pain with intercourse?
- Medical history
  - Are there any medical conditions that could be affecting reproductive success, for example, endocrine disorders such as thyroid disease or adrenal dysfunction?
  - Are chronic medical conditions such as asthma or diabetes in good control, or is there a need for optimization before fertility treatment?
  - What medications is the patient on, and do any of these needed to be discontinued or adjusted for someone trying to conceive?
- Surgical history
  - Does the patient have a prior surgery that involved or could have damaged the pelvis, for example, prior surgery for endometriosis or an appendectomy?
- Social history
  - What is the patient's smoking history?
  - Are there occupational exposures of concern, such as pesticides or radiation exposure?
  - Is the patient's relationship with her partner stable? How has the couple dealt with the stress of their infertility and has this affected intimacy?
- Family history
  - Is there any history of infertility in the family? How many siblings does the patient have, and does the timing between siblings suggest any delay in conception?
  - Is there any family history of thyroid disease, PCOS, obesity, or recurrent pregnancy loss (RPL)?
  - Is there any family history of breast or ovarian cancer?

The complete history should help to elucidate potential causes for the couples' infertility. Infrequent menses is suggestive of an ovulatory disorder and would prompt an endocrine evaluation. A past history of chlamydial infection or hospitalization for pelvic inflammatory disease would warrant an assessment of tubal status. Menorrhagia or intermenstrual spotting might indicate a submucosal fibroid or endometrial polyp. Thus, a careful history is the first step toward identifying potential issues with fertility.

Physical Examination

A physical examination can also help to identify factors that contribute to a couples' infertility. Focused physical examination for a woman with infertility would include the following assessment:

- General
  - Height/weight; both obesity and anorexia are associated with hormone abnormalities
  - Pulse; tachycardia or bradycardia may be present with thyroid disease
- Head and neck
  - Check thyroid for size, nodules, and tenderness
  - Assess for cervical, submandibular, or supraclavicular lymphadenopathy
- Breast
  - Examine for development (Tanner stage) and presence of masses or skin changes
  - Galactorrhea
- Abdomen
  - Assess for tenderness or masses
  - Examine for any surgical scars
- Pelvis
  - Check external genitalia for development as well as pubertal status (Tanner stage)
  - Speculum examination of vagina and cervix to assess for infections and anatomic abnormalities
  - Bimanual examination to assess uterine size, shape, and tenderness and for adnexal masses or tenderness
  - Rectovaginal examination to palpate for uterosacral nodularity or to further examine adnexa
- Skin
  - Hirsutism: check face, chest, and midline abdomen for extra hair growth
  - Acanthosis nigricans: typically present at nape of neck or in skin folds

Similar to the medical history, the physical examination will often uncover abnormalities that can explain a couples' difficulty in conceiving. For example, an obese woman with hirsutism and acanthosis nigricans may have PCOS as the underlying cause of her ovulatory disorder. A patient with dysmenorrhea and a tender adnexal mass may have endometriosis and an endometrioma. Physical examination findings are useful in pointing the infertility workup in the most likely direction.

Detection of Ovulation

Ovulation is an essential component of reproduction. The first half of the menstrual cycle is the follicular phase, when the pituitary gonadotropins follicle-stimulating hormone (FSH) and luteinizing hormone (LH) drive the development of a mature ovarian follicle. This follicle contains the oocyte and its surrounding granulosa and theca cells, and hormonal feedback from the follicle to the hypothalamus and pituitary culminates in the LH surge that results in ovulation. The luteal phase is the second half of the menstrual cycle that follows ovulation. During this 2-week period, steroid production by the ovarian follicle, now a corpus luteum, is progestin dominant rather than estrogen dominant to support a potential pregnancy. If implantation does not occur, the corpus luteum regresses, hormone levels drop, a withdrawal bleed occurs and a new cycle begins again.

The interplay of hormones in the hypothalamic-pituitary-ovarian axis that regulates the menstrual cycle can be disrupted, resulting in oligoovulation or anovulation. This disruption is reflected in menstrual irregularities, typically cycles of long duration or complete absence of cycles. The luteal phase is typically 14 days, whereas the follicular phase can be more variable. Most ovulatory cycles occur every 24 to 35 days, with ovulation occurring cycle day 10 to 21. There are several ways by which one can test for ovulation:

1. Menstrual calendar: A menstrual cycle that is normal in duration and frequency is highly suggestive of ovulation.
2. Urinary LH kits: These self-administered kits measure the LH surge that occurs midcycle.
3. Midluteal progesterone level: A cycle day 21 progesterone level greater than 3 ng/dL indicates ovulation. As progesterone release from the corpus luteum is pulsatile, further discrimination on the quality of ovulation based on progesterone level has not been found to be useful.

If menstrual cycles or other testing raises concern for an ovulatory disorder, it is reasonable to undertake an endocrine evaluation for further evaluation. Common causes of oligoovulation or anovulation include PCOS, thyroid disease, hypothalamic hypogonadism, hyperprolactinemia, and adrenal disease. Thus, laboratory work to evaluate for an ovulatory disorder includes the determination of the levels of the following:

- FSH
- LH
- Prolactin
- Thyroid-stimulating hormone
- Estradiol
- Androgens (total testosterone, dehydroepiandrosterone, 17-hydroxyprogesterone) if PCOS or nonclassical congenital adrenal hyperplasia are suspected

With these results, most endocrinopathies resulting in anovulation can be identified and therapy directed at correction of the underlying disorder. If none is identified, however, and the patient is confirmed to be anovulatory, ovulation induction with oral or injectable agents is still reasonable and is further discussed in the article by Propst elsewhere in this issue.

Evaluation of Tubal Status

Once an oocyte is released, it must be picked up by the fallopian tube and moved toward the uterus. Damage to the fallopian tube from infection, postsurgical adhesive disease, or endometriosis can disrupt function of the tubal fimbria and cilia. Fertilization typically occurs in the fallopian tube. Complete tubal obstruction will prevent fertilization, as sperm cannot reach the oocyte; partial tubal obstruction places the patient at risk of an ectopic pregnancy, as fertilization can occur but normal transport of the oocyte or embryo is disrupted.

Tubal status can be investigated by the following approaches:

1. Hysterosalpingogram (HSG): This fluoroscopic imaging study involves the injection of radiopaque dye through the cervix. The dye outlines the endometrial cavity, fills

the length of the fallopian tubes if the tubes are patent, and then spills into the pelvis potentially revealing pelvic adhesions if present.

2. Chromotubation: This procedure is performed during laparoscopy, whereby the dye is injected through the cervix and visualized spilling out of the fimbriated end of the tubes. This test may be used to confirm tubal blockage documented on HSG or in lieu of HSG in patients at increased risk for tubal disease such as those with prior pelvic infections or endometriosis.

3. Chlamydial antibody testing (CAT): This is a noninvasive serum test that identifies past chlamydial infections. This test is used to identify those at a greater risk of tubal adhesive disease and spare low-risk patients invasive testing.

There are advantages and disadvantages of each tubal investigation. The HSG provides imaging of the uterine cavity and tubes; however, it is purely a diagnostic test. Although it is thought that this flushing of the tubes can remove debris and increase the chance of conceiving, most abnormalities identified on HSG require additional evaluation and management by laparoscopy or pelvic ultrasonography. For this reason a laparoscopy may be a better choice for tubal evaluation of patients at high risk of tubal disease, as documentation of tubal patency and management of any tubal adhesive disease can be performed concomitantly, avoiding a second invasive procedure.

CAT is attractive as a noninvasive option of tubal assessment. *Chlamydia trachomatis* is a common pathogen in pelvic infections and some chlamydial infections are asymptomatic. The serum antibody test can be used to risk stratify patients for invasive tubal testing. If a patient has no risk factors for tubal disease and the CAT result is negative, an HSG can be deferred from the initial infertility workup. The CAT can pick up other chlamydial infections, such as *Chlamydia pneumoniae*, reducing the specificity of the test for pelvic disease.

A tubal evaluation is a critical part of the infertility workup because of the limited options for treatment if tubal disease is uncovered. Before the advent of in vitro fertilization (IVF), tubal surgery such as neosalpingostomies or tubal cannulation procedures were critical to those with obstructive disease. In current infertility practice, tubal surgery has a more restricted role because of the increasing success of IVF.[1]

Uterine Evaluation

The uterus, and specifically the endometrial layer, is important in reproduction as the site of implantation and fetal development. The uterus forms by fusion of the Müllerian ducts during early embryonic development. Failure of the ducts to fuse in the midline can result in congenital anomalies of the uterus that are associated with infertility, such as a uterine septum. Furthermore, with age, women can grow uterine fibroids or endometrial polyps that disrupt endometrial function and hamper implantation. Surgery on the uterus can result in scarring of the cervix or endometrial cavity.

Options for evaluation of the uterus and endometrial cavity include

1. HSG: As discussed previously, instillation of dye through the cervix outlines the endometrial cavity. This technique is sensitive for intracavitary or submucosal pathologic findings but may not pick up other uterine abnormalities such as intramural myomas.

2. Saline-infused sonohysterography (SIS): In this pelvic ultrasonography, a small catheter is used to instill sterile saline into the uterine cavity, allowing for a more sensitive evaluation of the uterine cavity and any potential pathologic finding.

3. Hysteroscopy: Direct visualization of the cavity either in the office or in the operative room setting can be used to assess for uterine abnormalities.

Although it is more certain that uterine adhesive disease or submucosal myomas can result in infertility and warrant surgical intervention, the impact of intramural myomas on fertility is more controversial.[2] Large intramural myomas that distort the endometrial cavity or have a submucosal component likely result in some impairment; smaller intramural or subserosal myomas likely have minimal impact on fecundity.

Attempts to test the integrity of the endometrial layer itself have not been successful. In the past, a routine part of the fertility evaluation included an endometrial biopsy to check for a luteal phase defect to ensure that follicular and endometrial tissue development was in synch. Studies have not shown this test to be a useful discriminator between the fertile and infertile populations, and it is no longer a recommended part of the infertility evaluation.[3] Investigation of other markers of endometrial receptivity such as β3-integrin has shown some promise but have yet to translate to improving clinical practice.[4]

Ovarian Reserve Testing

The link between the age and fertility of women is well known, with female fecundity starting to decline during the fourth decade and dropping more rapidly approaching and after age 40 years.[5] Pregnancy rates following donor oocyte IVF cycles reveal that treatment success is directed by the age of the oocyte donor rather than that of the recipient, demonstrating the impact of age on oocyte quality. It is established that the oocyte-related changes with age are not only quantitative but also qualitative. Oocytes accumulate meiotic errors over time, hence the greater incidence of aneuploidy in conceptuses and increased risk of miscarriages seen in older women.

"Ovarian reserve" refers to the measurement of both oocyte quality and quantity and should be performed in women who are older than 35 years or have a history or menstrual pattern that raises concern for diminished ovarian function. Traditionally, an early follicular (cycle day 2–4) FSH level has been used to test ovarian reserve, and FSH levels greater than 10 to 11 mIU/mL have been associated with diminished oocyte quality and infertility. The antral follicle count (AFC), a measurement of all 2- to 10-mm follicles in the early follicular phase, has also been shown to be a useful marker of ovarian reserve and predictor of fertility treatment success.[6] Serum anti-Müllerian hormone (AMH) is the newest marker of ovarian reserve and has the advantages of being cycle-independent and less subjective than the AFC. AMH is released by the granulosa cells of late preantral and small antral follicles and thus functions as a measurement of the remaining pool of follicles in the ovary.[7] It too has been shown to be predictive of fertility treatment success.[8,9]

Debate exists over the best marker of ovarian reserve. Each of the available options (**Box 4**) has been shown to be predictive of pregnancy; however, they likely measure different aspects of oocyte and ovarian follicular health. An FSH level more likely reflects hormonal integrity of the ovarian follicle, whereas the AFC and AMH more

---

Box 4
Ovarian reserve markers

- Age
- Follicle-stimulating hormone level
- Antral follicle count
- Anti-Müllerian hormone level

likely reflect the actual count of immature oocytes left in the ovary. In many cases, multiple markers are used concomitantly to estimate ovarian reserve. In the event of finding diminished ovarian reserve, referral to an infertility specialist is appropriate to allow for the use of more aggressive fertility treatments.

EVALUATION OF THE MALE PARTNER
Infertility History

It is estimated that male factor contributes to at least half of all infertile couples and is the sole cause of infertility in 15% to 20% of couples.[10] An evaluation of the male partner should be performed at the same time as the female partner and should also begin with a careful medical history.

- Reproductive history
  - Has the patient fathered pregnancies in the past?
  - Has he tried previously with another partner?
- Genitourinary history
  - Does the patient have a history of any penile or testicular disease, for example, undescended testicle?
  - Did he have any prior genital infections?
  - Does he have difficulty with maintaining erection or with ejaculation?
  - Was there trauma to the groin?
  - Is there a change in the size of the testes?
- Medical history
  - Are there any medical conditions that could affect sperm production, for example, recent febrile illnesses or chronic conditions?
  - What medications does the patient take, and could any of these impair sperm production or function (eg, exogenous testosterone)?
- Surgical history
  - Does the patient have a prior surgery that could impair genitourinary structures, for example, orchiectomy, inguinal hernia repair, or vasectomy?
- Social history
  - What is the patient's smoking history?
  - Are there occupational exposures of concern, such as pesticides or radiation exposure?
  - Is the patient's relationship with his partner stable? How has the couple dealt with the stress of their infertility, and has this affected intimacy?
- Family history
  - Is there any history of infertility in the family? How many siblings does the patient have, and does the timing between siblings suggest any delay in conception?

Similar to the clinical history of the female partner, the history of the male partner may uncover potential explanations for the couples' infertility. Exogenous testosterone use may be the cause of a reversible iatrogenic oligospermia, or past chemotherapy may have resulted in a permanent loss of sperm production. A family history of infertility may reveal an inheritable defect in sperm production. These findings help to direct additional workup and treatment.

Physical Examination

Physical examination of the male partner is typically performed by a urologist and is recommended for anyone with urogenital symptoms, symptoms of androgen deficiency, or abnormal semen analysis parameters. This examination includes the following:

- General
  - Height/weight, body habitus, and body mass
  - Secondary sex characteristics, such as facial hair
- Breast
  - Examine for gynecomastia
- Pelvis
  - Penile development and location of urethral meatus
  - Testicular volume and consistency
  - Presence of the vas deferens and assessment of epididymal induration
  - Palpation for a varicocele or hernia
  - Digital rectal examination if indicated

The examination of the male partner may reveal a lack of secondary sex characteristics, indicating hypogonadism, or absence of the vas deferens, which is a cause of obstructive azospermia. Although these findings would not be acted on without a semen analysis, this examination is an important part of the infertility workup when clinical history suggests a potential issue or to look for potentially reversible causes of abnormal semen analysis parameters.

Semen Analysis

Semen analysis is the cornerstone of male infertility evaluation. An ejaculate is collected, typically by masturbation, after a 2- to 7-day abstinence period and then evaluated by several parameters (**Table 1**). A sperm concentration of greater than 15 million/mL is normal, as is sperm motility of greater than 40%.[11] Forward progression is another method of scoring sperm motility, characterizing the movement of sperm as not only present but also directed. The morphology of sperm can be graded using careful measurements of the head and tailpiece; different morphologic criteria are used, such as the Kruger or World Health Organization (WHO) methods. Finally, ejaculate volume is used to assess for retrograde ejaculation or obstructive pathology.

Table 1 Semen analysis parameters	
Parameter	**Reference Values (Fifth Percentile)**
Ejaculate volume	1.5–5.0 mL
pH	>7.2
Sperm concentration	>15 million/mL
Total sperm number	>39 million/ejaculate
Motility	>40%
Forward progression	>32%
Morphology	>4% normal for Kruger >30% normal for WHO
Sperm agglutination	Absent
Viscosity	>2 cm thread postliquefaction

Data from World Health Organization. WHO laboratory manual for the examination of human semen and sperm-cervical mucus interaction. 3rd edition. Cambridge (United Kingdom): Cambridge University Press; 1992.

The pH of the sample should be alkaline as a result of the secretions from the seminal vesicles.

If an ejaculate is found to contain azospermia (no sperm), the sample must be centrifuged and the pellet resuspended and reexamined to ensure that there are no sperm. Further evaluation of a semen analysis includes an analysis of any additional cells seen, such as epithelial cells or leukocytes, as well as vitality stains for samples with poor motility. It is recommended that a patient with an abnormal semen parameter have at least 2 semen analyses performed to ensure consistency.

Additional Testing

For patients with abnormal semen parameters additional testing is indicated. In addition to a physical examination, an endocrine evaluation is recommended for any man with a sperm concentration of less than 10 million/mL. The hormones tested should include serum FSH and total testosterone; if the testosterone level is low in the setting of a low/normal FSH, prolactin and LH can also be measured. These laboratory findings should help differentiate gonadal failure from hypogonadism and also identify hyperprolactinemia.

If a low-volume ejaculate is seen, and is not due to collection error, possible causes include retrograde ejaculation or ejaculatory duct obstruction. To investigate retrograde ejaculation, a postejaculatory urinalysis is performed, and in the case of retrograde ejaculation sperm can be retrieved from the urine. If it is planned to use these sperm for fertility treatment, alkalinization of the urine before collection will improve sperm survival. Palpation of the vas deferens on examination and ultrasonography is performed to investigate ductal obstruction.

If severe oligospermia (<5 million/mL) is found and the physical examination does not reveal signs of obstruction, a genetic workup is appropriate to investigate an underlying genetic abnormality. A karyotype is recommended to look for aneuploidies such a Klinefelter syndrome (47,XXY) or a balanced translocation. Deletions specific to the Y chromosome that are associated with oligospermia have been identified. These Y-chromosome microdeletions in the azoospermia factor (AZF) region are more prevalent in men with infertility, and if present, the specific mutation can be prognostic of the success of a surgical sperm retrieval procedure.[12]

In cases of azospermia, a diagnostic testicular biopsy may be needed to procure sperm for fertility treatment. If found, sperm should be frozen to avoid the need for a second procedure. Furthermore, in cases in which a male partner has had a vasectomy, options are microsurgical tubal reversal versus surgical retrieval of sperm from the epididymis or testis to be used for IVF. Both are effective techniques; the success of tubal reversal does depend on the time elapsed since the initial vasectomy, with the best rates seen when the procedure is done within 15 years of the initial surgery.[13]

FUTURE DIRECTIONS

The field of infertility continues to evolve, and with this progress will come new techniques to evaluate couple with infertility. For the female partner, additional research is needed to understand the best way to measure ovarian reserve, and the development of different distension media for the SIS may allow for tubal status to be evaluated at the same time. For the male partner, current semen analysis is mainly descriptive, focusing on the count and appearance of sperm. Functional tests of sperm and testing of sperm DNA fragmentation may develop so that they become useful tests that enhance our understanding of male factor infertility and help to direct therapy.

SUMMARY

Infertility is a common condition afflicting couples and causes a considerable amount of distress. Infertility evaluation includes investigation of the female and male partners, with a careful history to identify potential issues; testing directed to assess ovulatory function and tubal status; and semen analysis. Additional testing beyond these basics can be pursued as indicated by the particular couples' history.

REFERENCES

1. Practice Committee of the American Society of Reproductive Medicine. Committee opinion: role of tubal surgery in the era of assisted reproductive technology. Fertil Steril 2012;97(3):539–45.
2. Practice Committee of the American Society of Reproductive Medicine and The Society of Reproductive Surgeons. Myomas and reproductive function. Fertil Steril 2008;90(Suppl 5):S125–30.
3. Coutifaris C, Myers ER, Guzick DS, et al. Histological dating of timed endometrial biopsy tissue is not related to fertility status. Fertil Steril 2004;82(5):1264–72.
4. Lessey BA. Assessment of endometrial receptivity. Fertil Steril 2011;96(3):522–9.
5. Committee on Gynecologic Practice of the American College of Obstetricians and Gynecologists, The Practice Committee of the American Society of Reproductive Medicine. Age-related fertility decline: a committee opinion. Fertil Steril 2008;90(Suppl 5):S154–5.
6. Hendriks DJ, Mol BW, Bancsi LF, et al. Antral follicle count in the prediction of poor ovarian response and pregnancy after in vitro fertilization: a meta-analysis and comparison with basal follicle-stimulating hormone level. Fertil Steril 2005; 83(2):291–301.
7. Ledger WL. Clinical utility of measurement of anti-mullerian hormone in reproductive endocrinology. J Clin Endocrinol Metab 2010;95(12):5144–54.
8. Hazout A, Bouchard P, Seifer DB, et al. Serum antimüllerian hormone/müllerian-inhibiting substance appears to be a more discriminatory marker of assisted reproductive technology outcome than follicle-stimulating hormone, inhibin B, or estradiol. Fertil Steril 2004;82(5):1323–9.
9. La Marca A, Sighinolfi G, Radi D, et al. Anti-Mullerian hormone (AMH) as a predictive marker in assisted reproductive technology (ART). Hum Reprod Update 2010;16(2):113–30.
10. Practice Committee of the American Society of Reproductive Medicine. Diagnostic evaluation of the infertile male: a committee opinion. Fertil Steril 2012; 98(2):294–301.
11. World Health Organization. WHO laboratory manual for the examination of human semen and sperm-cervical mucus interaction. 3rd edition. Cambridge (United Kingdom): Cambridge University Press; 1992.
12. Practice Committee of the American Society of Reproductive Medicine and the Society for Male Reproduction and Urology. Evaluation of the azoospermic male. Fertil Steril 2008;90(Suppl 5):S74–7.
13. Practice Committee of the American Society of Reproductive Medicine and the Society for Male Reproduction and Urology. The management of infertility due to obstructive azoospermia. Fertil Steril 2008;90(Suppl 5):S121–4.

Optimizing Natural Fertility
The Role of Lifestyle Modification

Mamie McLean, MD[a],*, Melissa F. Wellons, MD[b]

KEYWORDS

- Natural fertility • Preconception counseling • Obesity • Lifestyle modifications

KEY POINTS

- Preconception counseling allows health care providers to optimize maternal and neonatal outcomes before conception.
- Preconception counseling also provides a unique opportunity for health care providers to recommend, often simple, interventions to optimize natural fertility.
- Maternal obesity must be addressed during preconception counseling and include both patient education and recommendations regarding weight loss.
- The current body of literature examining lifestyle modifications and fertility is comprised of small cohort studies, most focus on polycystic ovarian syndrome, and use surrogate markers of fertility.
- Although the literature does support the improvement in ovulation and pregnancy rates with modest weight loss, the impact on live birth rates is not clear.
- Calorie restriction and exercise both seem to be beneficial in improving fertility; the optimal macronutrient content of a diet is not known.

INTRODUCTION

Human reproduction is notoriously inefficient, with average cycle fecundity averaging around 20%.[1] Preconception counseling allows physicians to help patients frame expectations for conception by reviewing baseline fecundity rates. Additionally, physicians can help educate patients on methods to optimize their natural fertility (**Box 1**), in the absence of, or concern for, pathologic conditions, before recommending aggressive interventions.

Perhaps more importantly, patients presenting for preconception counseling allow their physician to have a powerful platform to recommend interventions to improve

Disclosures: None.
[a] Division of Reproductive Endocrinology and Infertility, Department of Obstetrics and Gynecology, University of Alabama at Birmingham, 619 19th Street South, Room 10390 Women and Infants' Center, Birmingham, AL 35249-7333, USA; [b] Division of Medical Endocrinology, Department of Internal Medicine, Vanderbilt University, Nashville, TN, USA
* Corresponding author.
E-mail address: mamclean@uab.edu

Obstet Gynecol Clin N Am 39 (2012) 465–477
http://dx.doi.org/10.1016/j.ogc.2012.09.004
0889-8545/12/$ – see front matter © 2012 Published by Elsevier Inc.

obgyn.theclinics.com

> **Box 1**
> **American Society for Reproductive Medicine practice guidelines: optimizing natural fertility, 2008**
>
> - Fertility declines with age
>   - Women: 35 Men: 50
> - Frequency of Intercourse
>   - Intercourse every day to every other day yields highest cycle fecundability
> - 'Fertile Window'
>   - 6 day interval ending on the day of ovulation
>   - Peak fecundability when intercourse occurs within 2 days of ovulation
>   - Declines dramatically on the day of presumed ovulation
> - Monitoring Ovulation
>   - Cervical mucus functioned as well or better than basal body temperature or urinary LH monitoring
>   - Some evidence that LH detection kits decrease time to conception
> - Coital Practices
>   - No evidence that fecundability is affected by coital position
>   - Mineral oil, canola oil, hydroxyethylcellulose based lubricants do not adversely affect sperm motility
>   - Avoid water based lubricants (Astroglide®, KY Jelly®) due to affect on sperm motility
> - Smoking
>   - Increased risk of infertility, miscarriage
>   - Reduced time to menopause (1–4 years)
>   - Male fertility: smoking may decrease parameters in semen analysis
> - Alcohol
>   - No evidence that moderate consumption negatively impacts fertility
>   - Can affect fetal development, thus consumption should cease at first signs of pregnancy
> - Caffeine
>   - Moderate consumption (1–2 cups of coffee/day) has no adverse effects on fertility or pregnancy outcomes
> - Weight
>   - Over and underweight at risk for infertility and increased time to conception
>
> *Data from* Plymate SR, et al. Inhibition of sex hormone-binding globulin production in the human hepatoma (Hep G2) cell line by insulin and prolactin. J Clin Endocrinol Metab 1988;67(3):460–4.

overall health, in addition to improving maternal and neonatal outcomes before conception. The American Congress of Obstetrics and Gynecology (ACOG) has established clear recommendations for considerations during preconception counseling:

ACOG Preconception Guidelines 2005[2]
1. Evaluate preexisting, uncontrolled, or undiagnosed maternal diseases
2. Review prior obstetric history

3. Review vaccination history
4. Review medications, radiation exposure, and environmental hazards
5. Review mental health issues
6. Recommend folic acid 400 mcg/d or higher (4 mg/d) depending on risk factors
7. Evaluate family history and genetic risk.

In the setting of the obesity epidemic, physicians will be faced with an obese patient desiring conception. Although most patients and physicians are aware of the above recommendations for those seeking pregnancy, as well as the effect of weight on fertility, many physicians struggle when recommending a "prescription for weight loss."

The remainder of the article focuses on the available evidence regarding lifestyle modification (LSM) and fertility, and includes the aims listed in **Box 2**.

LSM improves fertility because it[3–11]

1. Decreases adipose tissue
    a. Improves insulin sensitivity
    b. Increases sex hormone–binding globulin (SHBG)
    c. Increases ovulatory cycles
    d. Improves pharmacodynamics of medications
    e. Improves hypothalamic function
2. Improves metabolic function of remaining adipose tissue
3. Reduces inflammation.

Although there is biologic plausibility for LSM improving fertility, there has not yet been confirmation in the literature. There are few well-controlled, randomized studies to date that have evaluated the effects of LSM specifically on fertility. Many of the studies that address reproductive function are small cohort studies or observational trials with no placebo group, high dropout rates, and surrogate markers for fertility.

OVULATION INDUCTION
Modest Weight Loss

Several studies have documented the resumption of ovulation after only modest weight loss of 5% to 10% of total body weight.

Crosignani and colleagues[12] found resumption in spontaneous ovulation with small reductions in overall body weight. These investigators placed 33 women with obesity, chronic anovulation, infertility, and polycystic ovaries on a 1200 kcal diet and recommended regular exercise. The women were evaluated once they reached 5% and

---

Box 2
Aims of article

1. Investigate the effects of LSM in obese women, including those with PCOS on the following reproductive outcomes:

    a. Ovulation rates

    b. Pregnancy rates

    c. Live birth rates

    d. ART success

2. Describe the available literature on the most effective diet and exercise regiments for improving fertility

10% total body weight loss. Twenty-five women lost at least 5% of their starting body weight and 11 women achieved 10% weight loss. Of the women who lost weight, 15 had resumption of ovulation. Among those women who did not lose the recommended weight, none experienced improvements in their menstrual cycles or conceived.

Only one study to date has studied obese, non-PCOS women. Clark and colleagues[13] completed an observational cohort study with 13 obese, clomiphene citrate (CC)-resistant women, including five with PCOS, with at least a 2-year history of infertility. PCOS and CC resistance were not clearly defined. All participants delayed conventional fertility treatments to participate in a 6-month diet and exercise program. After 4 months, the cohort had a mean weight loss of 4.3 kg and 92% of the group had achieved ovulation at that time, as demonstrated by urinary pregnanediol results.

Reduction in Centripetal Adipose Tissue

Centripetal adipose tissue is more metabolically active than subcutaneous adipose tissue and contributes more to insulin resistance.[14] Reductions in centripetal adipose tissue have been shown to (1) lower insulin resistance, (2) increase SHBG, and (3) potentially improve ovulation. Several studies have documented improved ovulation after reduction in centripetal adipose tissue (**Table 1**).

LSM and Response to CC

The traditional medication used to induce ovulation in women with eugonadotropic anovulatory infertility is CC. Success rates are as high as 80% but are lower for obese women.[15]

Palomba and colleagues[16] hypothesized that short LSM would improve response to medication. They conducted a randomized, controlled, single-blinded cohort study that involved 96 overweight or obese women with PCOS who were CC-resistant. Resistance was defined as failure to ovulate after a maximum dose of 150 mg of CC. The women were randomized to one of three groups for 6 weeks: (1) hypocaloric diet with structured exercise training (SET), (2) observation with CC, and (3) hypocaloric diet with SET and CC (combination). The primary outcome was rate of ovulation. The diet was high protein (35% protein, 45% carbohydrate, 20% fat) and adjusted to create a 1000 kcal deficit per day. The exercise training was three sessions per week, in 30-minute increments, on a bicycle ergometer, with the workload adjusted to 60% and 70% of maximal oxygen consumption. The combination group had the highest rate of ovulation at 37.5% compared with the hypocaloric diet and SET group at 12.5% and the CC alone group at 9.4%.

PREGNANCY RATES

Even obese women who are ovulatory demonstrate increased time-to-conception, which suggests detrimental effects of obesity on fertilization or implantation.[17]

Modest Weight Loss

Just as modest weight loss is beneficial for ovulation rates, a similar improvement is seen in pregnancy rates. In the hallmark study that evaluated LSM and fertility, Kiddy and colleagues[18] demonstrated improved fertility after modest weight loss. They evaluated 24 obese patients with PCOS and placed them on a 1000 kcal, low-fat diet for 6 to 7 months. Five of the 11 women who had ovulatory dysfunction at baseline conceived after losing more than 5% of their total body weight.

Table 1
LSM and central adipose tissue

Author	Design	Subjects	Intervention	Primary Outcome	Findings
Palomba et al,[21] 2008	Observational cohort	40 obese, infertile women with PCOS	24 wk structured exercise program (SET) vs diet SET = 3 times weekly exercise sessions on a bicycle ergometer for 30 min. with target VO2 60%–70% Diet = high protein (35% protein, 45% carbohydrate, 20% fat) and an 800 kcal total deficit per day	Pregnancy rate	No difference in PR When stratifying by intervention and by outcome: Ovulatory patients↓ waist circumference > non-ovulatory patients SET: −9.6 cm vs −2.5 cm $P<.05$; diet group: −9.4 cm vs −2.8 cm $P <.05$[18]
Thomson et al	RCT	94 obese women with PCOS	20 wk of one of the following: 1. Hypocaloric, high protein diet (DO) 2. Diet and aerobic exercise (DA) 3. Diet and aerobic/resistance training (DC)	Weight loss	Regardless of intervention, those who ovulated were more likely to have greater reductions in waist circumference and abdominal fat mass as determined by dual energy X-ray absorptiometry WC 13.4 vs 10.0 cm $P<.02$ and AbFM 0.5 vs 0.3 cm $P<.05$[1]
Huber-Buchholz et al,[8] 1999	Cohort	46 women with irregular menses	28 women received Group or individual diet and exercise counseling * 6 mo vs 18 controls	Ovulation	Women who ovulated after LSM were more likely to have reduced waist circumference and central abdominal fat than those that did not resume ovulation[11]
Kuchenbecker et al	Cohort	22 anovulatory, infertile women with PCOS	LSM program * 6 mo: Individualized exercise Hypocaloric diet (500 kcal/day deficit)	Ovulation	At three months, the ovulatory women were more likely to have lost more intra-abdominal fat by CT scan (12% vs 5% $P = .002$) These differences became even more pronounced when analyzed at 6 months. (18.5% vs 8.6% $P = .005$)[19]

Similarly, Crosignani and colleagues[12] found improved pregnancy rates in a group of anovulatory, infertile, obese women with weight loss of only 5% of their total body weight.

Galletly and colleagues[19] found similar improvements in pregnancy rates during fertility treatment after LSM in women who had modest weight loss (mean 6.2 kg ± 4.5 kg).

A reduction in serum insulin with an associated increase in SHBG is the proposed mechanism behind the improvement in pregnancy rates after modest weight loss. Hollmann and colleagues[20] demonstrated a pregnancy rate of nearly 30% after a 32-week LSM program in a cohort of obese, anovulatory patients after only modest weight loss. They related the improved pregnancy rates to improved glucose tolerance. Before the intervention, nearly 50% had impaired glucose tolerance; after LSM, only 4% had impaired glucose tolerance.

Palomba and colleagues[21] demonstrated improved glucose metabolism in their group of obese, infertile women with PCOS after 24 weeks of LSM. As described previously, the women were randomized to a SET program or to dietary intervention. The SET group had greater reduction in fasting insulin and SHBG than the dietary group did. Although no improvement in pregnancy rate was seen, due to high drop-out rate of 25%, they were unable to detect a significant difference between groups. However, the SET group did trend toward a higher pregnancy rate than the diet group did; 35% versus 10% ($P = .058$). Researchers hypothesized that the benefits of exercise in inducing skeletal muscle glucose metabolism resulted in these differences in insulin levels and, subsequently, the projected improvement in fertility.

LIVE BIRTH RATES

Obese women have lower live birth rates than age-matched normal weight controls owing to several factors, including increased risk of miscarriage.[22–24]

Also contributing to the reduced live birth rate is the association between obesity and aneuploidy and fetal anomalies.[25,26] Obese women are also more likely to develop pregnancy complications and are more likely to experience intrauterine fetal demise and early neonatal death, which also impact the live birth rate.[27,28] Discussion of these factors is beyond the scope of this article.

To date, only one study has evaluated the impact of LSM on live birth rates (**Box 3**).

ASSISTED REPRODUCTIVE TECHNOLOGIES

Most studies have not found that obesity impacts clinical pregnancy rates in assisted reproductive technology (ART) cycles. However, the largest study to date, from the SART CORS (Society for Assisted Reproductive Technology Clinic Outcomes Reporting System) database, demonstrated a significant impact of obesity. This retrospective cohort study of more than 45,000 embryo transfers found that increasing BMI was associated with higher odds of clinical pregnancy failure in women younger than 35-years-old, although BMI did not seem to affect donor oocyte cycles.[29] Other studies have found that increasing BMI is associated with poorer response to stimulation, as well as increased risk of cycle cancellation and treatment failure.[30,31]

Only one study to date has examined the effects of LSM and ART outcomes in a randomized fashion (**Box 4**).

CLINICAL RECOMMENDATIONS

Among the studies on fertility outcomes, a small number have compared interventions to determine the optimal diet and exercise regimen, few have compared diet to

---

Box 3
LSM and LBR

Clark and colleagues

- Expanded upon previous study
- Cohort of 87 women who had undergone the same lifestyle modification program for 6 mo
- 20 women dropped out
- Pre-program data is reported for comparison
- Average weight loss was 10.2 kg ± 4.3 kg
- After the program, the women went back to attempting conception
  - Spontaneously or with assistance via techniques ranging from ovulation induction to IVF/ICSI
- Regardless of the method of conception, those who remained in the program had higher pregnancy rates than those who dropped out
- Live birth rate = 67% after the program
- Miscarriage rate after the intervention dropped to 18% from 75% prior to starting the LSM. (P<.01)[5]

---

exercise, and even fewer have used clinically relevant reproductive outcomes to assess the efficacy of lifestyle modifications. National organizations have attempted to raise awareness among clinicians but guidelines are limited. The ACOG and the American Dietetic Association recognize the importance of prepregnancy weight loss for obese patients, but neither make specific recommendations about how to go about achieving this goal.[32,33]

Box 4
LSM and ART success

Moran and colleagues

- Pilot study on short term weight loss and IVF in an obese cohort with a BMI 28–45
- Randomized to active dietary intervention and exercise for 5–9 weeks or standard treatment prior to oocyte retrieval
  - Diet = hypocaloric and high protein
  - Exercise = home based conditioning with walking
- 46 women were randomized
  - 18 completed the active intervention, 20 completed the standard therapy
- Both groups had reductions in waist circumference
  - Intervention group had reduced weight and BMI
- No difference in pregnancy rate or live birth rate
  - Only powered to 38%
  - However, those who had reduction in waist circumference had a higher odds ratio of becoming pregnant. (OR 1.286 P = .042)[4]

DIET
Energy Restriction

The literature supports energy restriction as a method of improving metabolism and fertility. As noted above, Crosignani and colleagues[12] demonstrated improved ovulation rates and pregnancy rates with an energy-restricted diet. These investigators restricted calories per day by 800 to 1000.[18,20] However, there is no data regarding the optimal amount of caloric restriction and fertility.[34]

Macronutrient Content

There are few studies that evaluate fertility and diets using different macronutrients. In theory, diets with a low glycemic index or high in protein, which would improve insulin resistance, may be more effective in women with PCOS; however, this has not been supported by data.[34] Similarly, low carbohydrate diets would seem to be beneficial in obese women, but this diet has also not been shown to improve reproductive outcomes.

Moran and colleagues[35] randomized 45 obese women with PCOS to a high-protein diet (30% protein, 40% carbohydrate, 30% fat) or a low-protein diet (55% carbohydrate, 15% protein, 30% fat) and followed them for 16 weeks. There was no difference in weight loss or changes in body composition between diets. Additionally, there was no difference between the two diets in resumption of ovulation. However, due to a high dropout rate of 37%, the study was underpowered to detect a difference.

EXERCISE

The type, amount, and duration of exercise needed to improve reproductive outcomes are not known. The types of exercise programs included in LSM are widely varied in the literature regarding fertility, ranging from recommendations to increase physical activity to structured treadmill training with targeted oxygen consumption. However, the data from Clark and colleagues[13,36] underscores the potential significance of a SET intervention, including

- Improved ovulation rates, pregnancy rates, and live birth rates
- 1 hour of structured aerobic exercise per week, plus group therapy.

Only one study to date attempts to determine what method of exercise is the most beneficial in improving fertility (**Box 5**).

Diet Versus Exercise

Only two studies have examined the impact of diet versus exercise on defined reproductive outcomes.

Palomba and colleagues,[21] as described previously, randomized women to 24 weeks of either a SET program or a high-protein, hypocaloric diet. The SET group had higher ovulation rates, 24.8%, versus the diet group, 15.1% ($P = .032$), and no difference in pregnancy rates for the SET group, 6.2%, versus the diet group, 1.7% ($P = .075$); however, the study was underpowered. The ovulatory patients who were in the diet group lost more weight than the ovulatory SET patients. (-10.5 kg vs -5.6 kg, $P<.05$). To explain this finding, the investigators hypothesized that the exercise in the SET group enhanced skeletal muscle metabolism and, thus, improved glucose metabolism, as evidenced by the lower fasting insulin levels compared with the diet group (-23.4 vs -13.1, $P = <.05$). The improved insulin sensitivity would then increase ovulation and, thereby, improve pregnancy rates, despite less weight loss in the SET group. Although this study suggests the importance of exercise in an LSM program, it was not randomized, had no control group, and was underpowered.

Box 5
Method of exercise and fertility

Thomson and colleagues

- Randomized overweight and obese women with PCOS to:
  - Hypocaloric diet (DO)
  - Hypocaloric diet and aerobic exercise (DA)
  - Hypocaloric diet and aerobic-resistance exercise (DC)
  - Intervention = 20 weeks
- Weight loss was similar in all groups
  - Mean weight loss was 9.4 ± 1.9% of total body weight
- The two exercise groups had greater reductions in fat mass
  - Dual-energy x-ray absorptiometry
- The DA group had a greater number of ovulatory cycles
  - DA 3.10 ± 1.97, DO1.33 ± 1.63, DC 2.65 ± 1.70, P = .04[1]

A recently published randomized controlled trial, examined the effects of diet versus exercise on anthropometric indices and endocrine parameters. A secondary outcome was ovulation rate. Fifty-seven women with all three Rotterdam criteria for PCOS and a BMI greater than 27 were randomized to diet, exercise, or a diet and exercise group for 4 months. Fourteen patients dropped out, leaving 43 for analysis. Weight loss was more pronounced in the diet (-6%) and combination groups (-5%) than in the exercise group (-3%, $P<.05$). Ovulation was detected by midluteal progesterone in 15 out of 43 women. There was no significant difference between groups.[37]

Expert Opinion

Because the literature fails to provide clinicians with concrete, evidence-based recommendations; expert panels have attempted to fill in the gaps. The Androgen Excess and Polycystic Ovarian Syndrome Society (AEPCOS) focuses on obese women with PCOS and, in their position statement, notes the current paucity of data regarding clinical recommendations (**Box 6**).[38]

For obese women without PCOS, there are no specific recommendations, other than weight loss. Thus, the authors must extrapolate from the general population, and rely on the National Institute of Health recommendations for obese adults:

National Institute of Health and National Heart Lung and Blood Institute recommendations for weight loss
  - Hypocaloric diet, 500 to 1000 calorie deficit per day
  - Macronutrient composition: 50% to 60% carbohydrate, 26% fat, and19% protein
  - Moderate to vigorous physical activity for 60 minutes most days of the week.

Although the optimal diet and exercise regimen remains uncertain, what can be gathered from the literature is that the institution of a hypocaloric diet resulting in a reduction in weight of at least 5% to10%, impacts fertility. Exercise seems to help reduce visceral adipose tissue.

Box 6
LSM principles suggested for obesity management in PCOS

1. Lifestyle modification is the first form of therapy, combining behavioral (reduction of psychosocial stressors), dietary, and exercise management.

2. Reduced-energy diets (500–1000 kcal/day reduction) are effective options for weight loss and can reduce body weight by 7% to 10% over a period of 6 to 12 months.

3. Dietary pattern should be nutritionally complete and appropriate for life stage and should aim for <30% of calories from fat, <10% of calories from saturated fat, with increased consumption of fiber, fibre, whole-grain breads and cereals, and fruit and vegetables.

4. Alternative dietary options (increasing dietary protein, reducing glycemic index, reducing carbohydrate) may be successful for achieving and sustaining a reduced weight but more research is needed in PCOS.

5. The structure and support within a weight-management program is crucial and may be more important than the dietary composition. Individualization of the program, intensive follow-up and monitoring by a physician, and support from the physician, family, spouse, and peers will improve retention.

6. Structured exercise is an important component of a weight-loss regime; aim for >30 minutes per/day.

Reprinted from Fertility and Sterility. Vol 92, No 6. Moran L, Pasquali R, Teedle HJ, et al. Treatment of obesity in polycystic ovary syndrome: a position statement of the Androgen Excess and Polycystic Ovary Syndrome Society, 1966–1982, Copyright 2009; with permission from Elsevier.

SUMMARY

Patients seeking conception are often a highly motivated group and physicians are in a unique situation to make recommendations that may improve, not only maternal and neonatal outcomes, but, potentially, a woman's overall health and long-term morbidity and mortality.

ACOG and the American Society for Reproductive Medicine very clearly state the recommendations in terms of preconception counseling and the optimization of natural fertility; however, to date, no group has given a definitive endorsement of a specific LSM to improve fertility in the general population.

Certainly the silence from professional organizations is due to the current state of the literature regarding LSM and fertility. The studies that exist are small, without placebo groups, possess high drop-out rates, are often underpowered, and frequently do not include women with the highest BMIs. Minorities are also largely understudied in the area of LSM. Lifestyle modifications in women without PCOS is also absent from the literature.

Current literature supports the improvement of ovulation rates and pregnancy rates with only modest weight reduction and, specifically, interventions that target centripetal adiposity.

What is less clear is the relationship of LSM on live birth rates and ART cycles.

Preconception counseling should include a discussion of the negative impact of weight on maternal and neonatal outcomes; however, again, the magnitude of benefit from LSM on mitigating these conditions is not known. Research is needed on the most effective intervention for weight loss as well as the amount of weight loss necessary to impact reproductive outcomes.

The role of LSM on long-term, overall health is, perhaps, the real question. Does LSM limit weight gain over a person's life? Does LSM diminish the negative effects of weight on cardiovascular health and development of metabolic syndrome? Does LSM reduce mortality? If so, it is our duty as physicians to recommend these modifications to our young, otherwise healthy patients. Catching a captive audience, who desire fertility, and recommending modifications in lifestyle that could potentially impact reproductive success, as well as overall morbidity, mortality, and quality of life, is our obligation.

REFERENCES

1. Wilcox AJ, Weinberg CR, Baird DD. Timing of sexual intercourse in relation to ovulation. Effects on the probability of conception, survival of the pregnancy, and sex of the baby. N Engl J Med 1995;333(23):1517–21.
2. American College of Obstetricians and Gynecologists. ACOG Committee Opinion number 313, September 2005. The importance of preconception care in the continuum of women's health care. Obstet Gynecol 2005;106(3):665–6.
3. Plymate SR, et al. Inhibition of sex hormone-binding globulin production in the human hepatoma (Hep G2) cell line by insulin and prolactin. J Clin Endocrinol Metab 1988;67(3):460–4.
4. Pasquali R, et al. Characterization of obese women with reduced sex hormone-binding globulin concentrations. Horm Metab Res 1990;22(5):303–6.
5. Spritzer PM, et al. Leptin concentrations in hirsute women with polycystic ovary syndrome or idiopathic hirsutism: influence on LH and relationship with hormonal, metabolic, and anthropometric measurements. Hum Reprod 2001; 16(7):1340–6.
6. Pasquali R. Obesity and androgens: facts and perspectives. Fertil Steril 2006; 85(5):1319–40.
7. Vigorito C, et al. Beneficial effects of a three-month structured exercise training program on cardiopulmonary functional capacity in young women with polycystic ovary syndrome. J Clin Endocrinol Metab 2007;92(4):1379–84.
8. Huber-Buchholz M, Carey DG, Norman RJ. Restoration of reproductive potential by lifestyle modification in obese polycystic ovary syndrome: role of insulin sensitivity and luteinizing hormone. J Clin Endocrinol Metab 1999;84(4):1470–4.
9. Robker RL, Wu LL, Yang X. Inflammatory pathways linking obesity and ovarian dysfunction. J Reprod Immunol 2011;88(2):142–8.
10. Gleeson M, et al. The anti-inflammatory effects of exercise: mechanisms and implications for the prevention and treatment of disease. Nat Rev Immunol 2011;11(9):607–15.
11. Thompson D, et al. Physical activity and exercise in the regulation of human adipose tissue physiology. Physiol Rev 2012;92(1):157–91.
12. Crosignani PG, et al. Overweight and obese anovulatory patients with polycystic ovaries: parallel improvements in anthropometric indices, ovarian physiology and fertility rate induced by diet. Hum Reprod 2003;18(9):1928–32.
13. Clark AM, et al. Weight loss results in significant improvement in pregnancy and ovulation rates in anovulatory obese women. Hum Reprod 1995;10(10):2705–12.
14. Park HS, Lee K. Greater beneficial effects of visceral fat reduction compared with subcutaneous fat reduction on parameters of the metabolic syndrome: a study of weight reduction programmes in subjects with visceral and subcutaneous obesity. Diabet Med 2005;22(3):266–72.
15. Imani B, et al. Predictors of patients remaining anovulatory during clomiphene citrate induction of ovulation in normogonadotropic oligoamenorrheic infertility. J Clin Endocrinol Metab 1998;83(7):2361–5.

16. Palomba S, et al. Six weeks of structured exercise training and hypocaloric diet increases the probability of ovulation after clomiphene citrate in overweight and obese patients with polycystic ovary syndrome: a randomized controlled trial. Hum Reprod 2010;25(11):2783–91.

17. Gesink Law DC, Maclehose RF, Longnecker MP. Obesity and time to pregnancy. Hum Reprod 2007;22(2):414–20.

18. Kiddy DS, et al. Improvement in endocrine and ovarian function during dietary treatment of obese women with polycystic ovary syndrome. Clin Endocrinol (Oxf) 1992;36(1):105–11.

19. Galletly C, et al. Improved pregnancy rates for obese, infertile women following a group treatment program. An open pilot study. Gen Hosp Psychiatry 1996; 18(3):192–5.

20. Hollmann M, Runnebaum B, Gerhard I. Effects of weight loss on the hormonal profile in obese, infertile women. Hum Reprod 1996;11(9):1884–91.

21. Palomba S, et al. Structured exercise training programme versus hypocaloric hyperproteic diet in obese polycystic ovary syndrome patients with anovulatory infertility: a 24-week pilot study. Hum Reprod 2008;23(3):642–50.

22. Metwally M, et al. Does high body mass index increase the risk of miscarriage after spontaneous and assisted conception? A meta-analysis of the evidence. Fertil Steril 2008;90(3):714–26.

23. Lashen H, Fear K, Sturdee DW. Obesity is associated with increased risk of first trimester and recurrent miscarriage: matched case-control study. Hum Reprod 2004;19(7):1644–6.

24. Rittenberg V, et al. Influence of BMI on risk of miscarriage after single blastocyst transfer. Hum Reprod 2011;26(10):2642–50.

25. Stothard KJ, et al. Maternal overweight and obesity and the risk of congenital anomalies: a systematic review and meta-analysis. JAMA 2009;301(6):636–50.

26. Watkins ML, et al. Maternal obesity and risk for birth defects. Pediatrics 2003; 111(5 Part 2):1152–8.

27. Ovesen P, Rasmussen S, Kesmodel U. Effect of prepregnancy maternal overweight and obesity on pregnancy outcome. Obstet Gynecol 2011;118(2 Pt 1): 305–12.

28. Cedergren MI. Maternal morbid obesity and the risk of adverse pregnancy outcome. Obstet Gynecol 2004;103(2):219–24.

29. Luke B, et al. Female obesity adversely affects assisted reproductive technology (ART) pregnancy and live birth rates. Hum Reprod 2011;26(1):245–52.

30. Shah DK, et al. Effect of obesity on oocyte and embryo quality in women undergoing in vitro fertilization. Obstet Gynecol 2011;118(1):63–70.

31. Luke B, et al. The effect of increasing obesity on the response to and outcome of assisted reproductive technology: a national study. Fertil Steril 2011;96(4):820–5.

32. Siega-Riz AM, King JC. Position of the American Dietetic Association and American Society for Nutrition: obesity, reproduction, and pregnancy outcomes. J Am Diet Assoc 2009;109(5):918–27.

33. ACOG Committee on Gynecologic Practice. ACOG committee opinion. Number 319, October 2005. The role of obstetrician-gynecologist in the assessment and management of obesity. Obstet Gynecol 2005;106(4):895–9.

34. Anderson K, Norman RJ, Middleton P. Preconception lifestyle advice for people with subfertility. Cochrane Database Syst Rev 2010;(4):CD008189.

35. Moran LJ, et al. Dietary composition in restoring reproductive and metabolic physiology in overweight women with polycystic ovary syndrome. J Clin Endocrinol Metab 2003;88(2):812–9.

36. Clark AM, et al. Weight loss in obese infertile women results in improvement in reproductive outcome for all forms of fertility treatment. Hum Reprod 1998; 13(6):1502–5.
37. Nybacka A, et al. Randomized comparison of the influence of dietary management and/or physical exercise on ovarian function and metabolic parameters in overweight women with polycystic ovary syndrome. Fertil Steril 2011;96(6): 1508–13.
38. Moran LJ, et al. Treatment of obesity in polycystic ovary syndrome: a position statement of the Androgen Excess and Polycystic Ovary Syndrome Society. Fertil Steril 2009;92(6):1966–82.

Obesity and Reproductive Function

Emily S. Jungheim, MD, MSCI[a,*], Jennifer L. Travieso, BS[a],
Kenneth R. Carson, MD[b,c], Kelle H. Moley, MD[a]

KEYWORDS

- Fertility • Obesity • Reproduction • Public health

KEY POINTS

- There is an epidemic of obesity among women and men of reproductive age.
- Numerous epidemiologic and translational studies demonstrate adverse effects of obesity on various stages of the reproductive process, although the underlying mechanisms are largely unknown.
- Of all the evidence linking obesity to adverse reproductive function and outcomes, the most concerning is the evidence demonstrating links between preconceptional maternal obesity and long-term disease in the offspring.
- Weight loss through lifestyle interventions or surgical therapy may improve reproductive function and outcomes, but data are limited.
- Given the epidemic of obesity in women and men of reproductive age, efforts to understand the impact of obesity on reproductive function and outcomes are an important component of future public health policy.

MEASURING OBESITY AND REPRODUCTIVE RISK

Disentangling the individual components of obesity associated with poor health outcomes is difficult.[1,2] Body mass index (BMI), calculated as the weight in kilograms divided by the height in meters squared, or overall body size adjusted for height, is

Disclosures: This work was supported by grant K12HD063086 from the National Institutes of Health (NIH), Bethesda, Maryland. The contents of this work are the responsibility of the authors and do not necessarily represent the official views of the NIH.
[a] Division of Reproductive Endocrinology and Infertility, Department of Obstetrics and Gynecology, Washington University in St Louis, St Louis, MO, USA; [b] Division of Hematology and Oncology, Department of Internal Medicine, Washington University in St Louis, St Louis, MO, USA; [c] Division of Public Health Sciences, Department of Surgery, Washington University in St Louis, St Louis, MO, USA
* Corresponding author. Washington University in St Louis, Campus Box 8513, 4444 Forest Park Avenue, Suite 3100, St Louis, MO 63108.
E-mail address: jungheime@wustl.edu

obviously, the most accessible measure of obesity because tools for measuring BMI are readily available. On the other hand, adiposity (regional or total body fat), adipokine production, and lifestyle components may also contribute individually or together to the overall obesity-related health risk. The bulk of the work relating obesity to health risks has focused on chronic diseases; however, we are learning more about components of obesity that relate to reproductive risk.

Body Mass Index

In general, the risk of obesity-related reproductive morbidity is associated with increasing BMI. BMI categories are as follows:

- Overweight: 25 to 29.9 kg/m^2: increased disease risk
- Class I obesity: 30 to 34.9 kg/m^2: high disease risk
- Class II obesity: 30 to 34.9 kg/m^2: very high disease risk
- Class III obesity: 40 kg/m^2 or more: extremely high disease risk[3]

These standard BMI categories are born out of associations made between obesity and risks of developing chronic conditions such as diabetes and cardiovascular disease. Although these conditions may exist in some obese women of reproductive age, many of them have not had long enough exposure time to manifest these diseases. Instead, signs of poor reproductive function such as anovulation and/or subfertility may be the first obesity-related morbidity that younger women experience. Standard BMI categories were not developed to relate the risk that young women face of poor reproductive function. Despite this, BMI is the measure used most often in counseling obese women regarding reproductive and pregnancy risks. In fact, some providers and practice organizations advocate for restricting fertility treatment to women based on BMI.[4]

There may be more specific measures associated with reproductive risk in obese women because BMI represents a measure of total body energy balance. Recent translational work has demonstrated that better predictors of metabolic risk and disease may exist such as quantity of visceral adipose tissue and intrahepatic triglyceride content.[5] Also, epidemiologic work has shown strong associations between lifestyle factors such as diet and physical activity and risk of cardiovascular disease, both of which influence energy balance and BMI but are independent factors.[6,7] Whether or not there are markers of obesity-related reproductive risk better than BMI is yet to be determined. Further study of relationships existing among adipokines, various measures of adiposity, and lifestyle factors such as diet and physical activity and reproductive outcomes may prove useful. In the meantime, studies of reproductive risk and obesity that categorize risk by BMI represent most of the data that can be used clinically in counseling obese women.

Adipokines

Adipokines are signaling molecules produced by adipose cells, and their production varies with adipose mass. Adipokines that may be important to obesity-related morbidity include leptin, tumor necrosis factor α (TNF-α), interleukin 6 (IL-6), free fatty acids, and adiponectin.[8–10] Abnormalities in adipokines may cause inflammation and abnormal cell signaling, which in turn leads to impaired cellular metabolism and function.

Emerging evidence links abnormalities in adipokines to abnormal reproductive function.[8] For example, leptin may affect reproductive function at the level of the hypothalamus, providing the signal both to initiate reproductive maturation and to maintain normal signaling of the hypothalamic-pituitary-ovarian axis.[8,11] This mechanism has been demonstrated in a mouse model of diet-induced obesity in which hyperleptinemia causes central leptin resistance and hypogonadism.[11] Such a mechanism could explain findings of altered pulsatile luteinizing hormone (LH) amplitude in obese women.[12] Also, leptin and TNF-α levels vary between follicular and luteal phases of the menstrual cycle.[8] Although the significance of these variations in adipokines between the stages of the menstrual cycle is unknown, it is possible that they may affect signaling within the hypothalamic-pituitary-ovarian axis required for normal oocyte recruitment and ovulation. Other work has demonstrated that adiponectin signaling may be important to preimplantation embryonic development and implantation.[13] The authors have recently shown that elevated free fatty acid levels are associated with impaired oocyte maturation and decreased chances of pregnancy.[14,15] The specific role of various adipokines in reproductive function is largely unknown, but the aforementioned examples suggest that they may provide an important link between obesity and pathologic reproductive function.

Lifestyle: Dietary Factors

Dietary choices that contribute to obesity may also play a role in the adverse reproductive outcomes associated with obesity. The potential role of diet in reproductive function has been elegantly demonstrated through the Nurses Health Study II (NHSII), a prospective epidemiologic cohort study in which the lifestyle patterns of nurses are tracked and long-term health outcomes are followed up. In a series of publications, dietary choices, such as vegetable sources of protein as against animal proteins, and limiting the intake of transfats and refined carbohydrates have been shown to be associated with decreased risks of ovulatory infertility independent of the BMI and total caloric intake.[16–18] Work demonstrating that dietary changes improve ovulatory function in anovulatory obese women has yet to be done, but certainly, the prospective research that has come from NHSII on lifestyle and ovulatory infertility is intriguing and offers clinicians and their patients a place to institute lifestyle changes that may help with weight loss that does improve ovulatory function in obese women.[19]

Lipotoxicity is one mechanism by which fat intake may influence reproductive tissues.[20–24] This process is characterized by excess circulating long-chain saturated fatty acids, which are produced by adipocytes themselves and are also obtained through the diet. When the adipocytes can no longer store these fatty acids, other nonadipose cell types begin to store fat. This leads to an increase in the production of reactive oxygen species with subsequent mitochondrial dysfunction, endoplasmic reticulum stress, and ultimately, cell death.[25] The reproductive tissues affected include granulosa cells and oocytes, leading to impaired oocyte maturation and poor oocyte quality.[24,26] In a murine model, we have recently shown that brief preimplantation embryonic exposure to excess palmitic acid, a long-chain saturated fatty acid obtained from the diet and produced by adipocytes, can result in fetal growth restriction with subsequent postdelivery catch-up growth and a metabolic-like syndrome in adulthood.[21] Whether or not this work is representative of what happens in the human condition is unknown; however, it does suggest that preconceptional and periconceptional diet and obesity have long-term impact on the offspring.

Lifestyle: Physical Activity

Lack of physical activity decreases energy expenditure and contributes to developing and continuing obesity. Whether or not lack of activity and exercise directly contribute to the pathophysiologic mechanisms linking obesity to disease is unclear.[27] On the other hand, in another analysis using NHSII data that controlled for BMI, women with the highest levels of physical activity were less likely to have ovulatory infertility than women who had low levels of physical activity.[19] In another recent study of physical activity and time to pregnancy, increased physical activity levels were associated with decreased time to pregnancy.[28] Altogether, poor dietary choices and decreased levels of physical activity contribute to the development and sustenance of obesity,[27] and therefore, physical activity may be an important component to improve reproductive function in the setting of obesity.

A Culmination of Risk Factors: Adverse Reproductive Outcomes in Obesity

Anovulation

Increasing BMI and obesity are associated with increased reproductive risks including menstrual irregularities, typically a result of anovulation.[29] Metabolic abnormalities induced by obesity, such as insulin resistance, may promote the development of polycystic ovary syndrome (PCOS), a condition diagnosed by the presence of oligomenorrhea and hyperandrogenism; however, not all anovulatory obese women meet these diagnostic criteria. As discussed, adipokines may have effects on hypothalamic-pituitary signaling and communication that inhibit ovulation and thus pose another mechanism by which obesity may increase the risk of irregular menses and anovulation.[11,12] Different women may have a different threshold for anovulation at various different body weights and overall adiposity as hypothalamic-pituitary signaling depending on other environmental exposures and genetic factors.[30]

Subfertility

While anovulation certainly contributes to subfertility among obese women, even in obese women with regular cycles, the time to pregnancy is increased in this group compared with women of normal weight.[31] It has been argued this increase is due to decreased frequency of sexual intercourse among obese women; however, in a research done through the NIH-sponsored Reproductive Medicine Network's Pregnancy in Polycystic Ovary Syndrome Trial, obesity was not associated with decreased frequency of sexual intercourse in couples trying to conceive.[32] Whether or not subfertility in ovulatory obese women is secondary to poorer oocyte or embryo quality, impairments in embryo implantation, or a combination of all these factors is unknown.

Miscarriage

It is difficult to get a true measure of the risk of miscarriage among obese women who conceive spontaneously because many women with early pregnancy loss may not realize that they are pregnant and therefore may never present to their physicians. This situation may be especially true for obese women with irregular menses. On the other hand, studies of women undergoing fertility treatments offer a unique opportunity to capture preconceptional exposures such as obesity and to relate these preconceptional exposures to reproductive outcomes such as miscarriage and others including ovulation, time to pregnancy, pregnancy risks, and neonatal outcomes.[33] Despite the opportunity for preconceptional exposures that infertile women and women undergoing assisted reproductive technology (ART) offer for such measures, data from a recent meta-analysis of obesity and miscarriage risk demonstrate that in general obesity is associated with an increased risk of miscarriage; however, the evidence linking obesity to increased risk of miscarriage in women undergoing ARTs is insufficient.[34] It is possible that ART may counter the increased risks of miscarriage in the setting of obesity by allowing for selection of better embryos and therefore lower risk of miscarriage, by improving endometrial conditions through the supraphysiologic doses of gonadotropin administered, or by allowing for correction of abnormal oocyte metabolism through in vitro culture out of the abnormal environment that obesity poses. Data supporting these hypotheses are lacking.

Adverse pregnancy outcomes

In pregnancy, obesity is associated with significant increased risk of maternal and fetal morbidity including increased risk of preeclampsia, gestational diabetes, fetal growth abnormalities, stillbirth, congenital abnormalities, and the need for cesarean delivery.[35] This is also true for obese women who conceive with in vitro fertilization (IVF).[36]

The reproductive phenotype of obesity varies in its severity, as some women conceive without difficulty and proceed through pregnancy without complication, whereas others may have some or a combination of the reproductive outcomes discussed. At present, beyond measurements of BMI and history of preexisting diabetes, there are few reliable risk factors to predict which obese women are going to have adverse reproductive and pregnancy outcomes. Regardless of how minor the reproductive phenotype an obese woman expresses, emerging evidence that children of obese mothers are at increased risk of obesity-related morbidity later in life is concerning because we may be propagating the obesity-related health problems that are already common today in this so-called "Fifth Phase of the Epidemiologic Transition: The Age of Obesity and Inactivity."[37–40] The mechanisms leading to this increased risk of obesity in the offspring are unknown, but laboratory data from animal models suggest that maternal obesity imposes epigenetic changes that lead to obesity in the offspring.[20,41] Anticipated findings from the National Children's Study, an ongoing prospective cohort study of 100,000 children that includes collection of data regarding pregnancy exposures and development of chronic disease, may shed more light on these concerns.[42]

OBESITY'S REPRODUCTIVE TARGETS
The Central Nervous System (CNS)

As mentioned previously, obese women exhibit decreased LH pulse amplitude and decreased excretion of progesterone metabolites.[12] In addition to causing anovulation, abnormal LH pulsatility may affect ovarian follicular steroidogenesis, leading to abnormal oocyte recruitment and poor oocyte quality and/or altered endometrial development, and it could affect the function of the corpus luteum in the luteal phase. How decreased LH pulse amplitude specifically affects subsequent reproductive function has yet to be discerned, but in any case, it does highlight the fact that mechanisms leading to anovulation in obese women may be different from those leading to anovulation in nonobese women with PCOS.[30] We have demonstrated that ART outcomes in morbidly obese women with PCOS are worse than those in women with PCOS who are not morbidly obese, suggesting that it is not chronic anovulation alone or abnormal central nervous system (CNS) signaling that affects the ovarian follicle and subsequent reproductive function, but perhaps some other component of obesity that is also important.[43]

The Ovary, Ovarian Follicle, and Oocytes

The authors recently investigated the effects of diet-induced obesity in a reproductive mouse model.[20] They isolated ovaries from obese mice and nonobese controls and stained them for apoptosis. Ovaries taken from the obese mice demonstrated increased apoptosis in the cells of the ovarian follicles. Oocytes isolated from the obese mice were smaller, and fewer oocytes from these mice were mature compared with control mice. In another study using a diet-induced obesity model, Igosheva and colleagues[44] found that preconceptional obesity is associated with altered mitochondria in mouse oocytes and zygotes, possibly the result of oxidative stress. Obese mice were less likely to support blastocyst development compared with lean mice. The authors concluded that abnormal oocyte and early embryonic mitochondrial metabolism contribute to poor reproductive outcomes in obese women.

It could be that abnormal signaling from the CNS alone results in abnormal ovarian follicular recruitment and development with poor-quality oocytes in obese women; however, work done by Robker and colleagues[45] suggests otherwise. Dr Robker has demonstrated that insulin levels are increased in the ovarian follicular fluid isolated from obese women undergoing IVF compared with women of moderate weight. In further work using a diet-induced obesity model, Dr Robker has shown that a high-fat diet is associated with lipid accumulation in oocytes along with markers of a lipotoxic response.[22] Similarly, in specimens isolated from women undergoing IVF, the authors have demonstrated that increased ovarian follicular fluid free fatty acid concentrations are associated with poor oocyte quality.[14] Supporting the theory that dietary factors, adipokines, or some other circulating factors directly affect the ovarian follicle, granulosa cells exposed to increasing concentrations of palmitic acid, a long-chain saturated fatty acid obtained from the diet and made by adipocytes, undergo apoptosis with decreased hormone steroidogenesis.[46]

In addition to abnormal endocrine and paracrine cues along with circulating adipokines, inflammatory factors, and metabolites, other factors may play a role in ovarian follicular health. Citing evidence from in vitro models of ovarian follicular development and unpublished work demonstrating increased rigidity in ovaries from obese versus nonobese mice, Woodruff and Shea[47] hypothesize that the physical environment of the ovary may also contribute to the pathologic features of polycystic ovaries.

The Embryo

Abnormal metabolism and other oocyte quality issues may carry over into abnormal embryonic metabolism and competence. This has been demonstrated in animal models of type 1 diabetes, and is suspected to be important in the setting of obesity based on maternal models of diet-induced obesity.[20,48] Poor embryo quality may originate with the oocyte, but an abnormal tubal or uterine environment may also influence embryo quality. In an in vitro model of obesity, the authors exposed preimplantation embryos to excess amounts of palmitic acid—a fatty acid that has been detected in uterine and tubal fluid.[21] This exposure resulted in abnormal embryonic expression of the insulinlike growth factor (IGF-1) receptor, which is responsible for insulin signaling in the embryo. When transferred back into normal recipient mice, the palmitic-acid-exposed embryos resulted in growth-restricted fetuses and the offspring demonstrated a metabolic-like syndrome.[21] Data from a similar model of type II diabetes demonstrate that embryonic insulin resistance is associated with increased risk of miscarriage and that metformin, an insulin sensitizer, reverses this risk.[49] Obesity also induces insulin resistance and could potentially cause similar issues of insulin resistance in preimplantation embryos.[20] Whether or not embryonic insulin resistance underlies the increased risk of miscarriage seen among obese women is unknown, but there is evidence to suggest that treating women with recurrent miscarriages with metformin improves the chances of a live birth.[50] Randomized controlled trials supporting the routine use of metformin in obese women with recurrent pregnancy loss are lacking.

The Endometrium

The endometrium is yet another potential target of the abnormal milieu created by obesity. One model that has been used to specifically address the endometrium is the donor oocyte model. In this model, oocytes from healthy donors are transferred into women who are typically unable to conceive with their own oocytes. Researchers have evaluated the impact of increasing BMI of recipients of donor oocyte on embryonic implantation rate, clinical pregnancy rate, miscarriage rate, and chances of live birth. These studies have yielded conflicting results with several studies demonstrating a BMI-related impact on measures of reproductive success[51,52] and others demonstrating no effect.[53,54] In any case, however, alterations in endometrial gene expression in the peri-implantation period have been noted to be different in obese versus nonobese women.[55]

IMPROVING REPRODUCTIVE FUNCTION IN OBESE WOMEN WITH SUBFERTILITY
An Opportunity for Intervention

Obesity-related anovulation and subfertility may provide an important opportunity for preconceptional intervention and improvements in reproductive function and outcomes. These opportunities go beyond interventions for obesity because they include opportunities to screen for pregestational diabetes mellitus and optimization of glucose control in women who are diabetic, opportunities to screen for preconceptional rubella and varicella vaccination, counseling regarding healthy diet and lifestyle preconceptionally and during pregnancy including the use of prenatal vitamins, and screening for any other previously undiagnosed medical issues important to healthy pregnancy outcome such as thyroid disease.

Pregnancy has been referred to as a "teachable moment" for weight control and obesity prevention because it may motivate women to adopt improved lifestyle habits that may lead to better weight control.[56] It is agreed that efforts should be made to educate and counsel pregnant women about weight gain and a healthy lifestyle during pregnancy; however, for obese women, preconception interventions may offer more potential for an impact on subsequent reproductive and pregnancy outcomes than intragestational interventions.

Weight Loss Through Lifestyle Changes

There are little data regarding lifestyle changes in subfertile obese women and improvements in spontaneous conception and other reproductive outcomes. Most data that exist examine lifestyle changes in women with PCOS, and even these data are limited. In a recent Cochrane review on lifestyle intervention and PCOS, the effectiveness of lifestyle intervention in improving reproductive outcomes in women with PCOS was investigated.[57] The investigators limited their search to randomized controlled trials comparing lifestyle intervention to minimal or no treatment in women with PCOS and concluded that there were no existing data demonstrating an effect of lifestyle on clinical reproductive outcomes. The authors performed a systematic review of the literature to include observational studies eliminated by the Cochrane review and to include studies of obese women without PCOS. They searched Medline up to June 2012 using the keywords "weight loss" and "reproduction." The search was limited to studies in women published in English in the past 5 years. With this search,8 studies were identified. Of these, 6 studies investigated reproductive function after treatment with medical therapies including metformin, orlistat, sibutramine, and myo-inositol.[58–63] One study outlined the strategy of an ongoing trial evaluating the costs and effects of a structured lifestyle program in overweight and obese subfertile women in Norway, but no result was available.[64] Only 1 study reported specifically on the effects of a lifestyle intervention on reproductive function in obese women, and this was in obese women preparing to undergo IVF.[65] This study by Moran and colleagues[65] randomized 38 overweight and obese women to active dietary modification and exercise or standard treatment before IVF. The investigators found a significant effect of the intervention on BMI and weight but no difference in pregnancy or live births between the intervention group and control group. The sample size was small, which limited the outcomes investigated.

Clearly, further work investigating preconceptional weight loss and reproductive function is needed, particularly translational work investigating specific steps in the reproductive process so that improved treatments and evidence-based management can be developed for obese women hoping to conceive.

Weight Loss Through Bariatric Surgery

Clinically meaningful weight loss through lifestyle changes may be difficult for some women. Bariatric surgery may offer greater and more sustainable weight loss. In 2008, Maggard and colleagues[66] published a systematic review of pregnancy and fertility after bariatric surgery. The investigators found that women of reproductive age accounted for 49% of all patients undergoing bariatric surgery. Overall, they concluded that the data support improved pregnancy outcomes in women who have undergone bariatric surgery compared with obese women who have not undergone bariatric surgery. These outcomes included decreased risk of gestational diabetes and preeclampsia and improved neonatal outcomes. In their search, studies regarding fertility were limited. The investigators identified 6 observational studies published between 1988 and 2004. All these studies demonstrated improvement of menstrual cycles in women who underwent bariatric surgery, but none of the studies investigated fertility as a primary outcome.

To determine if additional studies had been published since the JAMA review regarding bariatric procedures and fertility, the authors performed a review of Medline up to June 2012, limiting studies to those performed in women and published in English in the past 5 years. Keywords searched were "bariatric surgery and reproduction." A total of 40 articles were identified, but 15 articles were reviews,[67–82] 16 were on pregnancy outcomes after bariatric surgery,[83–98] 3 were commentaries or author replies,[99–101] 2 investigated contraceptive use postbariatric surgery,[102,103] 1 was a cross-sectional assessment of reproductive health in women undergoing bariatric surgery,[104] 1 was a case report of empty follicle syndrome in a woman postbariatric surgery undergoing IVF,[105] and 1 article was a case series of IVF in women who had previously undergone bariatric surgery.[106] In these last two articles, special considerations were outlined for IVF in women with previous bariatric surgery.[106] Only 1 of the articles identified investigated reproductive function after bariatric surgery. In this article, Rochester and colleagues[107] discuss improvements in LH and progesterone metabolite excretion after weight loss in obese women who have undergone bariatric surgery.

COMPETING RISKS IN THE SETTING OF INFERTILITY: OBESITY VERSUS AGE

As discussed, for obese women with infertility, weight loss may offer improved fertility. On the other hand, after the age of 35 years, there may be less of an effect of obesity on fertility rates with IVF,[108,109] although the obstetric risks that obesity poses remain. Furthermore, after the age of 35 years, there is a decrease in success of IVF in all women undergoing IVF, regardless of the infertility diagnosis or BMI.[109] These issues make for a difficult clinical scenario because age and obesity become competing risks in treating women with infertility. Also, neither does preconceptional weight loss guarantee pregnancy nor does it guarantee a pregnancy and delivery free of complication. For these reasons, some women with infertility may choose to accept obesity-related risks and proceed with fertility treatment instead.

FERTILITY TREATMENT OF OBESE WOMEN

Numerous studies have demonstrated decreased efficacy of fertility treatments in obese women.[33,43] As a result, some centers offering fertility treatments have put BMI limits on who they will treat and what types of treatment they will offer. In fact, in New Zealand, where fertility treatments are covered under the national health care plan, there is a BMI cutoff of 32 kg/m^2 that limits access to IVF. In the United States, some fertility treatment centers have BMI restrictions; however, these restrictions vary from center to center and are not universally enforced.[110] Furthermore, despite decreased efficacy of fertility treatments, the success of various fertility treatment strategies still offer a reasonable chance of success in obese women.[43,111] Subsequently, members of the Ethics Committee of the American Society for Reproductive Medicine recently proposed that restricting access to fertility treatment based on BMI is discriminatory.[112]

THE NEED FOR TRANSDISCIPLINARY RESEARCH AND NOVEL APPROACHES

The authors propose that obesity research as it relates to reproduction requires a transdisciplinary approach because both obesity and reproduction are complex systems affected by social, environmental, biologic, economic, and genetic influences to name a few. Tackling the problem of reproduction in obese women will require cooperative efforts among experts in all these fields of study. Ultimately, this type of research may help inform models of shared decision making in which physicians and patients mutually decide how to proceed with strategies for fertility. These models may be especially helpful because there is a significant degree of uncertainty that exists in treating obese women with infertility.[113] Such models would likely include consideration of the potential risks and benefits an individual (at a given age and weight) would gain from fertility treatment with or without a strategy for weight loss before or during treatment.

SUMMARY

There are many components of obesity that may affect the different steps of the reproductive process leading to adverse reproductive outcomes. Clearly, there is good data demonstrating that weight loss improves ovulatory function in obese women and improves pregnancy outcomes. On the other hand, female fertility is limited by time, the reproductive phenotype of obesity is variable, and current measures of obesity are not reliable predictors of these phenotypes. Because of the complex nature of obesity and reproduction, when an obese woman with subfertility presents for fertility treatment, an individualized yet systematic approach is needed.

REFERENCES

1. Luke DA, Stamatakis KA. Systems science methods in public health: dynamics, networks, and agents. Annu Rev Public Health 2012;33:357–76.
2. Hammond RA. Complex systems modeling for obesity research. Prev Chronic Dis 2009;6(3):A97.
3. Clinical guidelines on the identification, evaluation, and treatment of overweight and obesity in adults–the evidence report. National Institutes of Health. Obes Res 1998;6(Suppl 2):51S–209S.
4. Balen AH, Anderson RA. Impact of obesity on female reproductive health: British Fertility Society, Policy and Practice Guidelines. Hum Fertil (Camb) 2007;10(4):195–206.

5. Fabbrini E, Magkos F, Mohammed BS, et al. Intrahepatic fat, not visceral fat, is linked with metabolic complications of obesity. Proc Natl Acad Sci U S A 2009; 106(36):15430–5.

6. Stampfer MJ, Hu FB, Manson JE, et al. Primary prevention of coronary heart disease in women through diet and lifestyle. N Engl J Med 2000;343(1):16–22.

7. Hu FB, Stampfer MJ, Manson JE, et al. Trends in the incidence of coronary heart disease and changes in diet and lifestyle in women. N Engl J Med 2000;343(8): 530–7.

8. Gosman GG, Katcher HI, Legro RS. Obesity and the role of gut and adipose hormones in female reproduction. Hum Reprod Update 2006;12(5):585–601.

9. Hampton T. Scientists study fat as endocrine organ. JAMA 2006;296(13): 1573–5.

10. Shuldiner AR, Yang R, Gong DW. Resistin, obesity and insulin resistance–the emerging role of the adipocyte as an endocrine organ. N Engl J Med 2001; 345(18):1345–6.

11. Tortoriello DV, McMinn J, Chua SC. Dietary-induced obesity and hypothalamic infertility in female DBA/2J mice. Endocrinology 2004;145(3):1238–47.

12. Jain A, Polotsky AJ, Rochester D, et al. Pulsatile luteinizing hormone amplitude and progesterone metabolite excretion are reduced in obese women. J Clin Endocrinol Metab 2007;92(7):2468–73.

13. Kim ST, Marquard K, Stephens S, et al. Adiponectin and adiponectin receptors in the mouse preimplantation embryo and uterus. Hum Reprod 2011;26(1):82–95.

14. Jungheim ES, Macones GA, Odem RR, et al. Associations between free fatty acids, cumulus oocyte complex morphology and ovarian function during in vitro fertilization. Fertil Steril 2011;95(6):1970–4.

15. Jungheim ES, Macones GA, Odem RR, et al. Elevated serum alpha-linolenic acid levels are associated with decreased chance of pregnancy after in vitro fertilization. Fertil Steril 2011;96(4):880–3.

16. Chavarro JE, Rich-Edwards JW, Rosner BA, et al. Dietary fatty acid intakes and the risk of ovulatory infertility. Am J Clin Nutr 2007;85(1):231–7.

17. Chavarro JE, Rich-Edwards JW, Rosner BA, et al. Protein intake and ovulatory infertility. Am J Obstet Gynecol 2008;198(2):210.e1–7.

18. Chavarro JE, Rich-Edwards JW, Rosner BA, et al. A prospective study of dietary carbohydrate quantity and quality in relation to risk of ovulatory infertility. Eur J Clin Nutr 2009;63(1):78–86.

19. Chavarro JE, Rich-Edwards JW, Rosner BA, et al. Diet and lifestyle in the prevention of ovulatory disorder infertility. Obstet Gynecol 2007;110(5):1050–8.

20. Jungheim ES, Schoeller EL, Marquard KL, et al. Diet-induced obesity model: abnormal oocytes and persistent growth abnormalities in the offspring. Endocrinology 2010;151(8):4039–46.

21. Jungheim ES, Louden ED, Chi MM, et al. Preimplantation exposure of mouse embryos to palmitic acid results in fetal growth restriction followed by catch-up growth in the offspring. Biol Reprod 2011;85(4):678–83.

22. Wu LL, Dunning KR, Yang X, et al. High-fat diet causes lipotoxicity responses in cumulus-oocyte complexes and decreased fertilization rates. Endocrinology 2010;151(11):5438–45.

23. Robker RL, Wu LL, Yang X. Inflammatory pathways linking obesity and ovarian dysfunction. J Reprod Immunol 2011;88(2):142–8.

24. Yang X, Wu LL, Chura LR, et al. Exposure to lipid-rich follicular fluid is associated with endoplasmic reticulum stress and impaired oocyte maturation in cumulus-oocyte complexes. Fertil Steril 2012;97(6):1438–43.

25. Schaffer JE. Lipotoxicity: when tissues overeat. Curr Opin Lipidol 2003;14(3): 281–7.
26. Wu LL, Norman RJ, Robker RL. The impact of obesity on oocytes: evidence for lipotoxicity mechanisms. Reprod Fertil Dev 2011;24(1):29–34.
27. Wolin KY, Carson K, Colditz GA. Obesity and cancer. Oncologist 2010;15(6): 556–65.
28. Wise LA, Rothman KJ, Mikkelsen EM, et al. A prospective cohort study of physical activity and time to pregnancy. Fertil Steril 2012;97(5):1136–1142.e1–4.
29. Obesity and reproduction: an educational bulletin. Fertil Steril 2008;90(Suppl 5): S21–9.
30. Fritz M, Speroff L. Clincal gynecologic endocrinology and infertility. 8th edition. Philadelphia: Lippincott Williams & Wilkins; 2011.
31. Wise LA, Rothman KJ, Mikkelsen EM, et al. An internet-based prospective study of body size and time-to-pregnancy. Hum Reprod 2010;25(1):253–64.
32. Pagidas K, Carson SA, McGovern PG, et al. Body mass index and intercourse compliance. Fertil Steril 2010;94(4):1447–50.
33. Jungheim ES, Moley KH. Current knowledge of obesity's effects in the pre- and periconceptional periods and avenues for future research. Am J Obstet Gynecol 2010;203(6):525–30.
34. Metwally M, Ong KJ, Ledger WL, et al. Does high body mass index increase the risk of miscarriage after spontaneous and assisted conception? A meta-analysis of the evidence. Fertil Steril 2008;90(3):714–26.
35. Catalano PM, Ehrenberg HM. The short- and long-term implications of maternal obesity on the mother and her offspring. BJOG 2006;113(10):1126–33.
36. Dokras A, Baredziak L, Blaine J, et al. Obstetric outcomes after in vitro fertilization in obese and morbidly obese women. Obstet Gynecol 2006;108(1):61–9.
37. Gaziano JM. Fifth phase of the epidemiologic transition: the age of obesity and inactivity. JAMA 2010;303(3):275–6.
38. Laitinen J, Jaaskelainen A, Hartikainen AL, et al. Maternal weight gain during the first half of pregnancy and offspring obesity at 16 years: a prospective cohort study. BJOG 2012;119(6):716–23.
39. Catalano PM, Hauguel-De Mouzon S. Is it time to revisit the Pedersen hypothesis in the face of the obesity epidemic? Am J Obstet Gynecol 2011;204(6):479–87.
40. Dabelea D, Crume T. Maternal environment and the transgenerational cycle of obesity and diabetes. Diabetes 2011;60(7):1849–55.
41. Dunn GA, Bale TL. Maternal high-fat diet effects on third-generation female body size via the paternal lineage. Endocrinology 2011;152(6):2228–36.
42. Landrigan PJ, Trasande L, Thorpe LE, et al. The National Children's Study: a 21-year prospective study of 100,000 American children. Pediatrics 2006;118(5): 2173–86.
43. Jungheim ES, Lanzendorf SE, Odem RR, et al. Morbid obesity is associated with lower clinical pregnancy rates after in vitro fertilization in women with polycystic ovary syndrome. Fertil Steril 2009;92(1):256–61.
44. Igosheva N, Abramov AY, Poston L, et al. Maternal diet-induced obesity alters mitochondrial activity and redox status in mouse oocytes and zygotes. PloS One 2010;5(4):e10074.
45. Robker RL, Akison LK, Bennett BD, et al. Obese women exhibit differences in ovarian metabolites, hormones, and gene expression compared with moderate-weight women. J Clin Endocrinol Metab 2009;94(5):1533–40.
46. Mu YM, Yanase T, Nishi Y, et al. Saturated FFAs, palmitic acid and stearic acid, induce apoptosis in human granulosa cells. Endocrinology 2001;142(8):3590–7.

47. Woodruff TK, Shea LD. A new hypothesis regarding ovarian follicle development: ovarian rigidity as a regulator of selection and health. J Assist Reprod Genet 2011;28(1):3–6.

48. Jungheim ES, Moley KH. The impact of type 1 and type 2 diabetes mellitus on the oocyte and the preimplantation embryo. Semin Reprod Med 2008;26(2): 186–95.

49. Eng GS, Sheridan RA, Wyman A, et al. AMP kinase activation increases glucose uptake, decreases apoptosis, and improves pregnancy outcome in embryos exposed to high IGF-I concentrations. Diabetes 2007;56(9):2228–34.

50. Moll E, Korevaar JC, Bossuyt PM, et al. Does adding metformin to clomifene citrate lead to higher pregnancy rates in a subset of women with polycystic ovary syndrome? Hum Reprod 2008;23(8):1830–4.

51. DeUgarte DA, DeUgarte CM, Sahakian V. Surrogate obesity negatively impacts pregnancy rates in third-party reproduction. Fertil Steril 2010;93(3):1008–10.

52. Bellver J, Melo MA, Bosch E, et al. Obesity and poor reproductive outcome: the potential role of the endometrium. Fertil Steril 2007;88(2):446–51.

53. Styne-Gross A, Elkind-Hirsch K, Scott RT Jr. Obesity does not impact implantation rates or pregnancy outcome in women attempting conception through oocyte donation. Fertil Steril 2005;83(6):1629–34.

54. Wattanakumtornkul S, Damario MA, Stevens Hall SA, et al. Body mass index and uterine receptivity in the oocyte donation model. Fertil Steril 2003;80(2): 336–40.

55. Bellver J, Martinez-Conejero JA, Labarta E, et al. Endometrial gene expression in the window of implantation is altered in obese women especially in association with polycystic ovary syndrome. Fertil Steril 2011;95(7):2335–41, 2341.e1–8.

56. Phelan S. Pregnancy: a "teachable moment" for weight control and obesity prevention. Am J Obstet Gynecol 2010;202(2):135.e1–8.

57. Moran LJ, Hutchison SK, Norman RJ, et al. Lifestyle changes in women with polycystic ovary syndrome. Cochrane Database Syst Rev 2011;(7):CD007506.

58. Metwally M, Amer S, Li TC, et al. An RCT of metformin versus orlistat for the management of obese anovulatory women. Hum Reprod 2009;24(4):966–75.

59. Ghandi S, Aflatoonian A, Tabibnejad N, et al. The effects of metformin or orlistat on obese women with polycystic ovary syndrome: a prospective randomized open-label study. J Assist Reprod Genet 2011;28(7):591–6.

60. Ladson G, Dodson WC, Sweet SD, et al. The effects of metformin with lifestyle therapy in polycystic ovary syndrome: a randomized double-blind study. Fertil Steril 2011;95(3):1059–1066.e1–7.

61. Gerli S, Papaleo E, Ferrari A, et al. Randomized, double blind placebo-controlled trial: effects of myo-inositol on ovarian function and metabolic factors in women with PCOS. Eur Rev Med Pharmacol Sci 2007;11(5):347–54.

62. Florakis D, Diamanti-Kandarakis E, Katsikis I, et al. Effect of hypocaloric diet plus sibutramine treatment on hormonal and metabolic features in overweight and obese women with polycystic ovary syndrome: a randomized, 24-week study. Int J Obes (Lond) 2008;32(4):692–9.

63. Panidis D, Farmakiotis D, Rousso D, et al. Obesity, weight loss, and the polycystic ovary syndrome: effect of treatment with diet and orlistat for 24 weeks on insulin resistance and androgen levels. Fertil Steril 2008;89(4):899–906.

64. Mutsaerts MA, Groen H, ter Bogt NC, et al. The LIFESTYLE study: costs and effects of a structured lifestyle program in overweight and obese subfertile women to reduce the need for fertility treatment and improve reproductive outcome. A randomised controlled trial. BMC Womens Health 2010;10:22.

65. Moran L, Tsagareli V, Norman R, et al. Diet and IVF pilot study: short-term weight loss improves pregnancy rates in overweight/obese women undertaking IVF. Aust N Z J Obstet Gynaecol 2011;51(5):455–9.
66. Maggard MA, Yermilov I, Li Z, et al. Pregnancy and fertility following bariatric surgery: a systematic review. JAMA 2008;300(19):2286–96.
67. Sarwer DB, Lavery M, Spitzer JC. A review of the relationships between extreme obesity, quality of life, and sexual function. Obes Surg 2012;22(4):668–76.
68. Conrad K, Russell AC, Keister KJ. Bariatric surgery and its impact on child-bearing. Nurs Womens Health 2011;15(3):226–33 [quiz: 234].
69. Wax JR, Cartin A, Wolff R, et al. Pregnancy following gastric bypass surgery for morbid obesity: maternal and neonatal outcomes. Obes Surg 2008;18(5):540–4.
70. Ginsburg ES. Reproductive endocrinology: pregnancy and fertility after bariatric surgery. Nat Rev Endocrinol 2009;5(5):251–2.
71. Guelinckx I, Devlieger R, Vansant G. Reproductive outcome after bariatric surgery: a critical review. Hum Reprod Update 2009;15(2):189–201.
72. Merhi ZO. Impact of bariatric surgery on female reproduction. Fertil Steril 2009; 92(5):1501–8.
73. Shah DK, Ginsburg ES. Bariatric surgery and fertility. Curr Opin Obstet Gynecol 2010;22(3):248–54.
74. Wax JR, Pinette MG, Cartin A, et al. Female reproductive issues following bariatric surgery. Obstet Gynecol Surv 2007;62(9):595–604.
75. Merhi ZO, Pal L. Effect of weight loss by bariatric surgery on the risk of miscarriage. Gynecol Obstet Invest 2007;64(4):224–7.
76. Kominiarek MA. Pregnancy after bariatric surgery. Obstet Gynecol Clin North Am 2010;37(2):305–20.
77. ACOG practice bulletin no. 105: bariatric surgery and pregnancy. Obstet Gynecol 2009;113(6):1405–13.
78. Shekelle PG, Newberry S, Maglione M, et al. Bariatric surgery in women of reproductive age: special concerns for pregnancy. Evid Rep Technol Assess 2008;(169):1–51.
79. Beard JH, Bell RL, Duffy AJ. Reproductive considerations and pregnancy after bariatric surgery: current evidence and recommendations. Obes Surg 2008; 18(8):1023–7.
80. Karmon A, Sheiner E. Pregnancy after bariatric surgery: a comprehensive review. Arch Gynecol Obstet 2008;277(5):381–8.
81. Abodeely A, Roye GD, Harrington DT, et al. Pregnancy outcomes after bariatric surgery: maternal, fetal, and infant implications. Surg Obes Relat Dis 2008;4(3): 464–71.
82. Landsberger EJ, Gurewitsch ED. Reproductive implications of bariatric surgery: pre- and postoperative considerations for extremely obese women of child-bearing age. Curr Diab Rep 2007;7(4):281–8.
83. Lesko J, Peaceman A. Pregnancy outcomes in women after bariatric surgery compared with obese and morbidly obese controls. Obstet Gynecol 2012; 119(3):547–54.
84. Stone RA, Huffman J, Istwan N, et al. Pregnancy outcomes following bariatric surgery. J Womens Health (Larchmt) 2011;20(9):1363–6.
85. Josefsson A, Blomberg M, Bladh M, et al. Bariatric surgery in a national cohort of women: sociodemographics and obstetric outcomes. Am J Obstet Gynecol 2011;205(3):206.e1–8.
86. Dell'Agnolo CM, Carvalho MD, Pelloso SM. Pregnancy after bariatric surgery: implications for mother and newborn. Obes Surg 2011;21(6):699–706.

87. Sheiner E, Edri A, Balaban E, et al. Pregnancy outcome of patients who conceive during or after the first year following bariatric surgery. Am J Obstet Gynecol 2011;204(1):50.e1–6.

88. Bebber FE, Rizzolli J, Casagrande DS, et al. Pregnancy after bariatric surgery: 39 pregnancies follow-up in a multidisciplinary team. Obes Surg 2011;21(10): 1546–51.

89. Carelli AM, Ren CJ, Youn HA, et al. Impact of laparoscopic adjustable gastric banding on pregnancy, maternal weight, and neonatal health. Obes Surg 2011;21(10):1552–8.

90. Santulli P, Mandelbrot L, Facchiano E, et al. Obstetrical and neonatal outcomes of pregnancies following gastric bypass surgery: a retrospective cohort study in a French referral centre. Obes Surg 2010;20(11):1501–8.

91. Lapolla A, Marangon M, Dalfra MG, et al. Pregnancy outcome in morbidly obese women before and after laparoscopic gastric banding. Obes Surg 2010;20(9): 1251–7.

92. Smith J, Cianflone K, Biron S, et al. Effects of maternal surgical weight loss in mothers on intergenerational transmission of obesity. J Clin Endocrinol Metab 2009;94(11):4275–83.

93. Sheiner E, Balaban E, Dreiher J, et al. Pregnancy outcome in patients following different types of bariatric surgeries. Obes Surg 2009;19(9):1286–92.

94. Dias MC, Fazio Ede S, de Oliveira FC, et al. Body weight changes and outcome of pregnancy after gastroplasty for morbid obesity. Clin Nutr 2009;28(2):169–72.

95. Weintraub AY, Levy A, Levi I, et al. Effect of bariatric surgery on pregnancy outcome. Int J Gynaecol Obstet 2008;103(3):246–51.

96. Wax JR, Cartin A, Wolff R, et al. Pregnancy following gastric bypass for morbid obesity: effect of surgery-to-conception interval on maternal and neonatal outcomes. Obes Surg 2008;18(12):1517–21.

97. Patel JA, Patel NA, Thomas RL, et al. Pregnancy outcomes after laparoscopic Roux-en-Y gastric bypass. Surg Obes Relat Dis 2008;4(1):39–45.

98. Ducarme G, Revaux A, Rodrigues A, et al. Obstetric outcome following laparo-scopic adjustable gastric banding. Int J Gynaecol Obstet 2007;98(3):244–7.

99. Macones GA, Stamilio DM, Odibo A, et al. Discussion: 'bariatric surgery and obstetric outcomes' by Josefsson. Am J Obstet Gynecol 2011;205(3):e1–2.

100. Rinaldi AP, Kral JG. Comments on Sheiner et al's "Pregnancy outcome of patients who conceive during or after the first year following bariatric surgery". Am J Obstet Gynecol 2011;205(4):e11 [author reply: e11–2].

101. Devlieger R, Vansant G, Guelinckx I. Bariatric surgery. Am J Obstet Gynecol 2011;205(3):e7 [author reply: e7–8].

102. Mody SK, Hacker MR, Dodge LE, et al. Contraceptive counseling for women who undergo bariatric surgery. J Womens Health (Larchmt) 2011;20(12): 1785–8.

103. Paulen ME, Zapata LB, Cansino C, et al. Contraceptive use among women with a history of bariatric surgery: a systematic review. Contraception 2010;82(1): 86–94.

104. Gosman GG, King WC, Schrope B, et al. Reproductive health of women electing bariatric surgery. Fertil Steril 2010;94(4):1426–31.

105. Hirshfeld-Cytron J, Kim HH. Empty follicle syndrome in the setting of dramatic weight loss after bariatric surgery: case report and review of available literature. Fertil Steril 2008;90(4):1199.e21–3.

106. Doblado MA, Lewkowksi BM, Odem RR, et al. In vitro fertilization after bariatric surgery. Fertil Steril 2010;94(7):2812–4.

107. Rochester D, Jain A, Polotsky AJ, et al. Partial recovery of luteal function after bariatric surgery in obese women. Fertil Steril 2009;92(4):1410–5.
108. Sneed ML, Uhler ML, Grotjan HE, et al. Body mass index: impact on IVF success appears age-related. Hum Reprod 2008;23(8):1835–9.
109. Luke B, Brown MB, Stern JE, et al. Female obesity adversely affects assisted reproductive technology (ART) pregnancy and live birth rates. Hum Reprod 2011;26(1):245–52.
110. Harris ID, Python J, Roth L, et al. Physicians' perspectives and practices regarding the fertility management of obese patients. Fertil Steril 2011;96(4): 991–2.
111. Koning AM, Mutsaerts MA, Kuchenbecher WK, et al. Complications and outcome of assisted reproduction technologies in overweight and obese women. Hum Reprod 2012;27(2):457–67.
112. Bryzyski R, Fox J, Zera C, et al. Weight limits for access to fertility services: discriminatory or nonmaleficence? 2011.
113. Politi MC, Han PK, Col NF. Communicating the uncertainty of harms and benefits of medical interventions. Med Decis Making 2007;27(5):681–95.

Polycystic Ovarian Syndrome Management Options

G. Wright Bates Jr, MD[a],*, Anthony M. Propst, MD[b]

KEYWORDS

- Polycystic ovarian syndrome • Clomiphene citrate • Metformin
- Ovarian dysfunction

KEY POINTS

- The diagnosis of polycystic ovarian syndrome (PCOS) requires hyperandrogenemia, hirsutism, and/or polycystic ovarian morphology.
- Lifestyle modifications with structured exercise and diet programs are key to reducing the metabolic and reproductive dysfunction associated with PCOS.
- Metformin is the first-line agent for glucose intolerance associated with PCOS and may play a role as an adjunct to ovulation induction therapies.
- Clomiphene citrate (CC) remains the first line for oral ovulation induction. Letrozole's potential role in ovulation induction for women with PCOS seems promising but awaits definite data.
- Injectable gonadotropins increase the potential for ovulation but require intensive monitoring to avoid higher-order multiple pregnancies and ovarian hyperstimulation syndrome.
- Ovarian drilling should be reserved for women who fail medical management.
- Careful attention to health maintenance with assessment of cardiovascular and cancer risk is required in this patient population.

INTRODUCTION

Stein and Leventhal[1] are often credited with publishing the first article describing PCOS in 1935. Since their description of women with ovarian enlargement and absence of menses more 80 years ago, PCOS has garnered considerable attention and now may be the most common endocrine disorder, affecting up to 15% of all reproductive-aged women, depending on the diagnostic criteria used.[2] The

Dr Propst is a Colonel in the United States Air Force Medical Corps. The opinions and conclusions in this article are those of the authors and are not intended to represent the official position of the Department of Defense, United States Air Force, or any other government agency.

[a] Department of Obstetrics and Gynecology, University of Alabama School of Medicine, 619 19th Street South, Building 176F, Room 10390, Birmingham, AL 35249-7333, USA; [b] Department of Obstetrics and Gynecology, Uniformed Services University of the Health Sciences, 4301 Jones Bridge Road, Bethesda, MD 20814, USA
* Corresponding author.
E-mail address: wbates@uab.edu

Obstet Gynecol Clin N Am 39 (2012) 495–506
http://dx.doi.org/10.1016/j.ogc.2012.10.001
0889-8545/12/$ – see front matter © 2012 Elsevier Inc. All rights reserved.

reproductive sequalae of PCOS reflect ovarian dysfunction with the failure of antral follicles to develop into mature follicles. The cardinal signs of PCOS are enlarged ovaries with multiple small ovarian follicles and hyperandrogenism, often associated with hirsutism and metabolic syndrome. Obesity and glucose intolerance are common components of the PCOS clinical picture. Although there is no definitive laboratory test to confirm PCOS, the current consensus is to use a combination of symptoms and signs to diagnose PCOS.

DIAGNOSIS

PCOS spans a wide spectrum of reproductive and metabolic disorders. Women with PCOS may present with scant facial hair and irregular menses in an otherwise healthy state or have profound effects, such as absent menses, a full beard, severe insulin resistance, and morbid obesity, often seen with the hyperandrogenism, insulin resistance, and acanthosis nigricans syndrome.[3] This heterogeneity adds to the controversy surrounding the diagnosis of this syndrome. More than 2 decades ago, the National Institutes of Health convened a consensus conference to develop formal diagnostic criteria for PCOS.[4] The original criteria included

- Clinical or biochemical evidence of hyperandrogenism
- Chronic anovulation
- Exclusion of other known disorders

These criteria were updated by the Rotterdam European Society of Human Reproduction and Embryology (ESHRE)/American Society for Reproductive Medicine (ASRM) PCOS consensus workshop group.[5,6] This gathering concluded that PCOS is a syndrome of ovarian dysfunction along with the cardinal features of hyperandrogenism and polycystic ovary (PCO) morphology. The Rotterdam criteria are the most commonly used guidelines for the diagnosis of PCOS and require 3 of the following 4:

- Irregular or absent ovulation defined as 8 or fewer menstrual cycles per year
- Clinical (hirsutism) or biochemical (raised serum testosterone levels) signs of androgen excess
- Polycystic-appearing ovaries with 12 or more antral follicles ranging in size from 2 mm to 9 mm and increased ovarian volume of at least 10 mL^3 (**Fig. 1**)

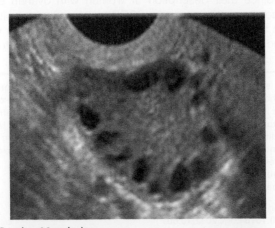

Fig. 1. Polycystic Ovarian Morphology.

AND

- Exclusion of other causes, including congenital adrenal hyperplasia (CAH), androgen-secreting tumors, and Cushing syndrome

Conversely, the Androgen Excess and PCOS Society states that PCOS should be first and foremost viewed as a syndrome of androgen excess.[7] They stress that PCOS is not a specific disease but a syndrome with a group or collection of signs (physical findings) and symptoms (patient complaints) that suggest a common disorder. Their diagnostic criteria include

- Hyperandrogenism with hirsutism and/or elevated free testosterone

AND

- Ovarian dysfunction with oligoanovulation and/or polycystic ovaries

AND

- Exclusion of other androgen excess or related disorders

The slight variability among these diagnostic criteria allow for many clinical presentations. It has been estimated that up to 10 distinct phenotypes are possible based on the different combinations of the 4 clinical symptoms: hyperandrogenemia, hirsuitism, menstrual dysfunction, and polycystic ovarian morphology.[7]

Polycystic ovarian morphology provides the namesake of this condition and can be visualized on transvaginal ultrasound in the majority of women with this syndrome. Most experts argue, however, that the presence of polycystic ovaries in the absence of androgen excess and ovarian dysfunction does not warrant the diagnosis of PCOS. Women with marked elevation of androgens or rapid onset of clinical symptoms may require imaging to screen for an androgen secreting neoplasm. Transvaginal ultrasound assessment of the endometrial cavity may be warranted in some women with PCOS to detect uterine hyperplasia or cancer.

Before the diagnosis of PCOS is made, other endocrine disorders should be considered. All anovulatory patients should be screened for hypothyroidism and hyperprolactinemia. In the presence of acne, hirsutism, or virilization, testing for androgen excess should be done. In PCOS, a normal to mildly elevated level of androgens is expected; however, excessive levels of testosterone or dehydroepiandrosterone sulfate (DHEAS) could indicate an androgen-producing tumor in the adrenal gland or ovary.

Clinically, it can be difficult to distinguish PCO from CAH because they both can have hirsutism and anovulation. CAH is usually caused by 21-hydroxylase deficiency. The screening test for CAH is 17-OH progesterone, which is elevated in CAH.

Cushing syndrome, a rare disorder with an incidence of 10 to 15 people per million, may also present with menstrual regularities and infertility.[8] The highest risk groups are patients with poorly controlled diabetes, hypertension, and early-onset osteoporosis. Testing is recommended in patients with multiple symptoms and signs of Cushing syndrome, including a round (or moon) face, buffalo hump on the back of the neck, abdominal obesity, and abdominal striae. Patients with Cushing syndrome usually have hypertension and glucose intolerance. The syndrome is caused by chronic exposure to excess glucocorticoids. A 24-hour urine cortisol or overnight dexamethasone suppression test is the preferred screening test for Cushing syndrome. Cushing disease refers to one specific cause of Cushing syndrome, a tumor in the pituitary gland that produces large amounts of corticotropin, which in turn elevates cortisol.

CLINICAL PRESENTATION

Women with PCOS present with a wide range of symptoms. The most common are menstrual irregularities[7]; 80% of women have menstrual irregularities, ranging from the more common oligomenorrhea to the less common amenorrhea. Oligomenorrhea usually results from anovulatory estrogen breakthrough bleeding after a prolonged period without ovulation to produce endogenous progesterone. Most women with PCOS have polycystic ovaries on ultrasound (75%–90%) and biochemical or clinical signs of androgen excess (70%). The androgen excess is manifested by hirsutism (60%–75%) and, more rarely, male pattern balding. Women with PCOS are commonly obese (65%–75%) and also frequently have insulin resistance (50%–70%). PCOS is also one of the most frequently seen causes of infertility and the most common cause of ovulatory dysfunction, present in 70% of women with ovulatory dysfunction.[9]

There is considerable overlap between PCOS and the metabolic syndrome but the two are not synonymous. The metabolic syndrome is present, however, in 30% to 40% of the women with PCOS and many of the individual components (truncal obesity, hypertension, and hyperlipidemia) are even more common.[10] Many of the metabolic manifestations of PCOS can be attributed to hyperinsulinemia.[11] Insulin resistance in tissues leads overproduction of insulin and results in hyperinsulinemia. This hyperinsulinemia is not purely related to obesity because women with PCOS are more likely to have insulin resistance than weight-matched controls. Hyperinsulnemia act on the liver to suppress sex hormone–binding globulin (SHBG) production. As SHBG is decreased, the levels of circulating free androgens increases. Not only does hyperinsulinemia decrease SHBG but it also stimulates pituitary luteinizing hormone (LH) production, which increases androgen production by the ovaries (**Fig. 2**). Researchers continue to explore the pathophysiologic mechanism underlying the spectrum of disease seen with PCOS, but the reproductive and metabolic dysfunction associated with this syndrome warrants a comprehensive approach.

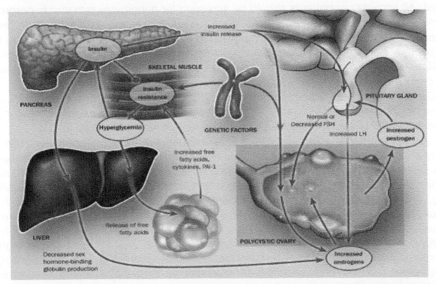

Fig. 2. Polycystic Ovarian Syndrome Pathophysiology. (*Adapted from* Nestler JE. Metformin for the treatment of the polycystic ovary syndrome. N Engl J Med 2008;358(1):47–54).

TREATMENT OPTIONS
Lifestyle Modification

Among women with PCOS, 65% to 75% are obese. Obesity has a significant impact on reproductive outcome. When a woman's body mass index (BMI) is greater than 35, the time to conception is increased 2-fold to 4-fold. Obesity not only influences time to conception but also adversely affects the response to fertility treatment. It also plays a role in adverse pregnancy outcomes once pregnant. There is an increased risk of miscarriage, congenital anomalies, and third-trimester pregnancy complications, in particular, preeclampsia and stillbirth.[12] Women should be provided with assistance to lose weight, including psychological support, dietary advice, exercise classes, and, where appropriate, weight-reducing agents or bariatric surgery.

The recommended first line of treatment is weight loss. Randomized control trials have found that weight loss strategies that use in-person support or remote support (telephone, e-mail, Web site) are more effective in achieving and sustaining clinically significant weight loss than patients whose weight loss is self-directed.[13] Studies have also shown that women with PCOS who initiate lifestyle changes with dietary changes, physical activity, and behavioral advice have lower levels of hirsutism, hyperandrogenism, weight and waist circumference, and insulin resistance.[14] A study evaluating patients with PCOS doing a structured exercise program averaging 92 minutes per week reported an average 5% reduction in BMI and 60% resumption of normal menses.[15] Palomba and colleagues[16] examined structured exercise programs compared with hypocaloric hyperprotein diets in women with PCOS and found the group that had a structured exercise program had significantly higher frequency of ovulation and spontaneous menses. Both the exercise group and the diet group had significantly lower weights, BMI, waist circumference, insulin resistance indexes, and serum levels of SHBG, androstenedione, and DHEAS compared with baseline. They also found that patients with PCOS who failed to ovulate when given 100 mg of CC for 5 days (CC resistant), had significantly higher rates of ovulation when given CC after 2 weeks of a structured exercise program and low caloric diet, compared with those who did not change their diet or exercise.[17]

Medical Management of PCOS

Weight loss

A wide array of complementary alternative medicines and prescription drugs have been proposed to combat the obesity and metabolic dysfunction associated with PCOS. Although acupuncture may be viewed as a surgical intervention, some investigators have suggested that it reduces hyperandrogenism and improves menstrual frequency in PCOS.[18] Americans also spend millions of dollars on diet aids despite few data on their efficacy. A recent systematic review concluded that nonprescription dietary supplements as an adjunct to weight loss currently cannot be strongly recommended.[19] Prescription weight loss medications also suffer from nebulous efficacy data and often concerning side-effect profiles. The only therapy currently Food and Drug Administration approved for the long-term management of obesity, orlistat, may be effective for the glucose intolerance associated with PCOS because it has been shown to reduce BMI and the progression to type 2 diabetes mellitus. Its use is limited, however, by gastrointestinal side effects.[20] Recent data support the use of phentermine/topiramate in obese and overweight adults. This drug combination has been shown to reduce weight, decrease cardiovascular risk factors, and improve metabolic function when used in conjunction with lifestyle modification.[21] These medications, however, have not been adequately assessed in women with PCOS and should be avoided in anyone pursuing fertility.

Hormonal suppression

Many women who do not desire fertility present to their health care provider complaining of the menstrual irregularity, hirsutism, or acne associated with PCOS. Oral contraceptives (OCPs) are the first-line therapy for most of these women. In addition to menstrual cycle regulation, OCPs reduce LH-mediated androgen production and decrease the biologic activity of androgens by increasing SHBG. Antiandrogens, including spironolactone, flutamide, and finasteride, have equivalent efficacy for hirsutism but have not been shown to augment the benefit seen with OCPs. New hair growth may also be reduced with topical therapy, eflornithine hydrochloride.[22] Despite the available of many agents to combat excess hair growth, removal techniques, including laser and electrolysis, are preferable in many circumstances.

The Amsterdam ESHRE/ASRM-sponsored thirrd PCOS consensus workshop group summary recommendation for the medical management of symptoms associated with androgen excess and PCOS included

- The benefits of OCPs outweigh the risks in most patients with PCOS and subsequent fertility is not reduced.
- There is no evidence for differences in effectiveness for contraception and hirsutism or risks among the various progestogens and when used in combination with a 20-mg versus a 30-mg daily dose of estrogen.
- Prolonged (>6 months) medical therapy for hirsutism is necessary to document effectiveness.
- Antiandrogens should not be used without effective contraception.
- Flutamide is of limited value because of its dose-dependent hepatotoxicity.

Ovulation induction

PCOS is the most common cause of ovulatory dysfunction and one of the most frequently seen identifiable causes of infertility. CC is the most common initial oral ovulation induction medication. CC is taken 3 to 5 days after the onset of a spontaneous or progestin induced menses.[23] Treatment typically begins with a single 50-mg tablet daily for 5-day and is increased by 50 mg up 250 mg a day in subsequent months if ovulation cannot be confirmed. Most conceptions occur within the first 6 ovulatory cycles and at doses of less than 150 mg a day but the fecundity rate decreases dramatically with age (<4% at >41 years of age).[24,25] Letrozole is an aromatase inhibitor that is used off label for ovulation induction in women who fail to conceive with CC. Letrozole is typically prescribed at a starting dose of 2.5 mg to 5 mg and can be increased by increments of 2.5 mg but the optimum dose range has not been established.[26] Letrozole may have a better side-effect profile and result in fewer multiple pregnancies. Definitive data regarding efficacy and unsubstantiated concerns for potential birth defects limit its adoption as a first-line agent. Ovulation induction is discussed at length in the article by Propst elsewhere in this issue.

Metformin

Metformin is a biguanide antihyperglycemic agent approved for the treatment of type 2 diabetes mellitus. It decreases blood glucose levels by suppressing hepatic glucose levels, decreasing intestinal absorption of glucose, and enhancing the peripheral glucose uptake and use.[27] When used in anovulatory women with PCOS, it acts to decrease insulin levels and LH. As the levels of insulin and LH are decreased, the level of SHBG increases. Ultimately, the levels of androgens are decreased, in part because of the increased level of SHBG but also because LH decreases. Women with PCOS also benefit from metformin because it typically causes a slight reduction in weight.[28–30] One study showed a 16% reduction in weight, resulting in a 200% increase in glucose clearance in women taking metformin.[31]

Studies have found that approximately 50% of women with PCOS or anovulatory cycles resume regular menses after taking metformin for 6 months. This is also true in adolescents with PCOS; many resume regular menses 4 to 6 months after initiating therapy with metformin.[27]

The target dose of metformin, in anovulatory patients, is typically 1500 mg to 2500 mg. The most common side effects are gastrointestinal in nature and include diarrhea, nausea, emesis, flatulence, indigestion, and abdominal discomfort. The reported discontinuation rate is 5% secondary to side effects.[27] Metformin XL or the liquid formation typically has fewer side effects.[32] Metformin is excreted by the kidney and can be linked to lactic acidosis in women with renal insufficiency or liver dysfunction. It should be temporarily suspended before surgery or radiologic procedures that use intravenous (IV) contrast.[27]

Metformin is a category B drug for pregnancy. The preliminary studies of women with PCO who continue metformin in pregnancy show that it may lower the incidence of first trimester losses and reduce the development of gestational diabetes. There have been no documented adverse effects on birth weight, growth, or motor development through 18 months of development.[33,34]

Metformin and clomiphene citrate

The combination of metformin and CC seems to have an additive effect in some anovulatory women. In Nestler and colleagues' landmark study, 60 PCOS women with a mean BMI of 32.3 were randomized to metformin (500 mg 3 times daily) versus placebo.[35] Women who did not ovulate on metformin or placebo were given CC 50 mg days 5 to 9; 90% of the obese, PCOS women who received metformin plus CC ovulated whereas 8% of the women who received CC plus placebo ovulated.

Metformin has also been compared head-to-head with CC for ovulation induction in anovulatory women with PCOS. In an Italian study of women with PCOS and a BMI less than 30, the incidence of ovulation with CC or metformin was examined.[36] The rates of ovulation were similar between the 2 groups, at approximately 65%. The pregnancy rates (PRs) were higher, however, in the metformin arm at (70%) compared with CC arm (34%), whereas the miscarriage rates were higher in the CC arm. This study first suggested that metformin may be a better first-line treatment of ovulation induction for women with PCOS.

A more comprehensive, multicenter National Institutes of Health–sponsored study looked at the live birth rates (LBRs) in more than 600 women with PCOS and oligoovulation or anovulation who were randomized to up to 6 months of treatment with CC alone, metformin alone, or a combination of CC and metformin.[37] The LBR was 22.5% in the CC group, 7.2% in the metformin group, and 26.8% in the group receiving metformin and CC. The LBR was significantly higher in women taking either CC alone or in the combination group, confirming that CC is a superior first-line treatment for anovulatory women with PCOS.

A recent meta-analysis of 14 prospective trials also showed a reduction in the LBR in the group of patients treated with metformin as a first-line agent when compared with CC alone (odds ratio [OR]= 0.48; 95% CI, 0.31–0.73; P = .0006). It also found an increase in ovulation (OR 1.6; 95% CI, 1.2–2.1; P = .0009) and PR (OR 1.3; 95% CI, 1.0–1.6; P = .05) in patients treated with a combination of CC and metformin compared with CC alone, but no difference was found when LBR was analyzed (OR 1.1; 95% CI, 0.8–1.5; P = .61).[38]

A 3-month course of metformin before initiating infertility treatment, however, seems to improve LBRs when compared with a placebo. A recently published multicenter trial in Finland randomized 320 women with PCOS and anovulatory infertility equally to metformin (BMI $\geq$27 mg/m^2 received 2000 mg daily; BMI <27 mg/m^2 received 1500 mg daily) or placebo.[39] After 3 months' treatment, another appropriate infertility treatment was combined if necessary. Intent-to-treat analysis showed that metformin significantly improved PR and LBR (vs placebo) in the whole study population (PR 53.6 vs 40.4%, P = .006; LBR 41.9 vs 28.8%, P = .014) and PR in women with a BMI greater than or equal to 27 mg/m^2 (49.0 vs 31.4%, P = .04) with a trend toward improved LBR (35.7 vs 21.9%, P = 0.07). Cox regression analysis showed that metformin plus standard infertility treatment increased the chance of pregnancy 1.6 times (95% CI, 1.13–2.27). In summary, women with a BMI greater than or equal to 27 mg/m^2 especially seem to benefit from 3 months' pretreatment with metformin before initiating ovulation induction and this can be combined with lifestyle changes in women who are trying to lose weight.

Surgical Management of PCOS

Before the availability of ovulation induction agent, surgical intervention was the gold standard for the treatment of PCOS. The enlarged polycystic ovaries were initially believed the cause of the androgen excess and reproductive dysfunction and, thus, amenable to surgical intervention. Removal of a wedge of the ovarian by laparotomy often resulted in restoration of ovulation in 8 of 10 women and PRs that exceeded 50%. The improvements in ovarian function, however, were often temporary and fertility potential reduced by adhesion formation.[40] The development of minimally invasive surgery, including laparoscopy, has led to a resurgence of interest in the surgical interventions for PCOS.

Laparoscopic ovarian diathermy (LOD) is a contemporary version of the Stein-Leventhal ovarian wedge resection for PCOS. It is a laparoscopic procedure in which electocautery or laser is used to create focal areas of damage in the ovarian cortex to reduce circulating and intraovarian androgen levels and reduce the volume of ovarian stroma. Approximately 4 to 20 areas of damage are created. It has the most success in women with a BMI less than 30 and an LH of greater than 10.

LOD is recommended by expert consensus as a second-line intervention, as are gonadotropins, in women with PCOS who are CC resistant.[41] The use of exogenous gonadotropins is associated with increased risk for a multiple pregnancy and requires intense monitoring of ovarian response. LOD is a good choice for those women for whom gonadotropin therapy is not practical due to long distances from a fertility specialist or those patients who have economic or religious concerns with using gonadotropins. LOD alone is usually effective in less than 50% of women and additional ovulation induction medication is required when the surgery itself does not result in spontaneous ovulation.[41,42]

LOD has been compared with CC as a first-line intervention and found less effective in a randomized clinical trial.[42] There is a risk of adhesions or ovarian damage after ovarian diathermy. LOD has also been compared with metformin in women with PCOS who did not ovulate with CC treatment.[43] This randomized controlled trial looked at ovulation, pregnancy, miscarriage, and LBRs between the two groups. The rates of ovulation after LOD or metformin (850 mg twice a day) were not statistically different. The PRs (18.6% vs 13.4%), miscarriage rates (15.4% vs 29%), and LBRs (82.1% vs 64.5%) were statistically better in the metformin group.

A recent Cochrane review evaluated 9 trials involving LOD, including 1210 women.[22] Live births were reported in 34% of women in the LOD group and 38% in the medically treated groups, including CC, letrozole, and gonadotropins. The LOD group had significantly fewer live births (OR 0.44; 95% CI, 0.03–0.52; P = .004) compared with the CC plus metformin subgroup. The rate of multiple pregnancies was significantly lower in the LOD group compared with trial using gonadotropins (OR 0.13; 95% CI, 0.03–0.52; P = .04).

HEALTH MAINTENANCE

Patients with PCOS are at risk for metabolic syndrome, diabetes, or cardiovascular disease and it is imperative that health care providers perform appropriate screening. The Androgen Excess and PCOS Society states that risk-category women with PCOS who also display obesity (especially abdominal adiposity), cigarette smoking, hypertension, dyslipidemia (increased low-density lipoprotein cholesterol [LDL-C] and/or non–high-density lipoprotein cholesterol [HDL-C]), subclinical vascular disease, insulin or glucose intolerance, and a family history of premature CVD (<55 years of age in male relative or <65 years of age in female relative) undergo the following screening:

- Blood pressure, waist circumference, and BMI at every visit
- Lipid profile (total cholesterol, LDL-C, non–HDL-C, HDL-C, and triglycerides) every 2 years
- 2-Hour post–75-g oral glucose challenge performed with a BMI greater than 30 kg/m^2 or, alternatively, in lean PCOS women with advanced age (>40 years), personal history of gestational diabetes, or family history of type 2 diabetes mellitus

The 3rd PCOS consensus workshop group recommended CVD risk assessment at any age for psychosocial stress, blood pressure, glucose, lipid profile (cholesterol, triglycerides, HDL, LDL, and non–HDL-C), waist circumference, physical activity, nutrition, and smoking.[2]

Screening for depression, anxiety, and quality of life[44] as well as sleep apnea[45] has also been suggested. Menstrual irregularity and obesity may also warrant heightened surveillance with endometrial biopsy or uterine ultrasound for endometrial cancer in women with PCOS.

SUMMARY RECOMMENDATIONS

- Lifestyle modifications with diet and exercise with weight loss are key to the successful management of both the reproductive and metabolic dysfunction seen in association with PCOS.
- Metformin, 1500 mg to 2500 mg daily, may be used in conjunction with CC in women with PCOS who do not ovulate when using CC alone. It is less efficient when used alone compared with CC for ovulation induction but may be beneficial when initiated alone for 3 months in overweight and obese women who are trying to lose weight before starting ovulation induction medications.
- Oral ovulation agents are the first-line treatment for ovulatory infertility seen with PCOS.
- Injectable gonadotropins may result in higher-order multiples and, thus, require thoughtful consideration of the risk/benefit profile with careful monitoring.
- LOD is a second-line intervention that is less effective than the combination of CC and metformin. It may be indicated for patients with fail to ovulate with oral agents for whom gonadotropins are a poor choice due to distance from fertility specialists or concern about a multiple pregnancy.

- Routine health maintenance and proper screening for metabolic syndrome, diabetes, and cardiovascular disease are crucial in the proper care of women with PCOS.

REFERENCES

1. Stein RI, Leventhal M. Amenorrhea associated with bilateral polycystic ovaries. Am J Obstet Gynecol 1935;29:181–5.
2. Fauser BC, Tarlatzis BC, Rebar RW, et al. Consensus on women's health aspects of polycystic ovary syndrome (PCOS): the Amsterdam ESHRE/ASRM-Sponsored 3rd PCOS Consensus Workshop Group. Fertil Steril 2012;97(1):28–38.e25.
3. Barbieri R, Ryan K. Hyperandrogenism, insulin resistance, and acanthosis nigricans syndrome: a common endocrinopathy with distinct pathophysiologic features. Am J Obstet Gynecol 1983;147(1):90–101.
4. Zawadski JK, Dunaif A. Diagnostic criteria for polycystic ovary syndrome: towards a rational approach. In: Dunaif A, Givens JR, Haseltine FP, et al, editors. Polycystic ovarian syndrome. Boston: Blackwell Scientific Publications; 1992. p. 377–84.
5. Rotterdam ESHRE/ASRM-Sponsored PCOS consensus workshop group. Revised 2003 consensus on diagnostic criteria and long-term health risks related to polycystic ovary syndrome (PCOS). Hum Reprod 2004;19(1):41–7.
6. Practice Committee of the American Society for Reproductive Medicine. Use of clomiphene citrate in women. Fertil Steril 2006;86(5 Suppl 1):S187–93.
7. Azziz R, Carmina E, Dewailly D, et al. The Androgen Excess and PCOS Society criteria for the polycystic ovary syndrome: the complete task force report. Fertil Steril 2009;91(2):456–88.
8. Guaraldi F, Salvatori R. Cushing syndrome: maybe not so uncommon of an endocrine disease. J Am Board Fam Med 2012;25(2):199–208.
9. ACOG Committee on Practice Bulletins–Gynecology. ACOG Practice Bulletin No. 108: polycystic ovary syndrome. Obstet Gynecol 2009;114(4):936–49.
10. Ehrmann DA, Liljenquist DR, Kasza K, et al. Prevalence and predictors of the metabolic syndrome in women with polycystic ovary syndrome. J Clin Endocrinol Metab 2006;91(1):48–53.
11. Nestler JE. Metformin for the treatment of the polycystic ovary syndrome. N Engl J Med 2008;358(1):47–54.
12. Balen AH, Anderson RA. Impact of obesity on female reproductive health: British Fertility Society, Policy and Practice Guidelines. Hum Fertil (Camb) 2007;10(4): 195–206.
13. Appel LJ, Clark JM, Yeh HC, et al. Comparative effectiveness of weight-loss interventions in clinical practice. N Engl J Med 2011;365(21):1959–68.
14. Moran LJ, Hutchison SK, Norman RJ, et al. Lifestyle changes in women with polycystic ovary syndrome. Cochrane Database Syst Rev 2011;(7):CD007506.
15. Vigorito C, Giallauria F, Palomba S, et al. Beneficial effects of a three-month structured exercise training program on cardiopulmonary functional capacity in young women with polycystic ovary syndrome. J Clin Endocrinol Metab 2007;92(4): 1379–84.
16. Palomba S, Giallauria F, Falbo A, et al. Structured exercise training programme versus hypocaloric hyperproteic diet in obese polycystic ovary syndrome patients with anovulatory infertility: a 24-week pilot study. Hum Reprod 2008; 23(3):642–50.
17. Palomba S, Falbo A, Giallauria F, et al. Six weeks of structured exercise training and hypocaloric diet increases the probability of ovulation after clomiphene

citrate in overweight and obese patients with polycystic ovary syndrome: a randomized controlled trial. Hum Reprod 2010;25(11):2783–91.

18. Raja-Khan N, Stener-Victorin E, Wu X, et al. The physiological basis of complementary and alternative medicines for polycystic ovary syndrome. Am J Physiol Endocrinol Metab 2011;301(1):E1–10.

19. Poddar K, Kolge S, Bezman L, et al. Nutraceutical supplements for weight loss: a systematic review. Nutr Clin Pract 2011;26(5):539–52.

20. Derosa G, Cicero AF, D'Angelo A, et al. Effects of 1-year orlistat treatment compared to placebo on insulin resistance parameters in patients with type 2 diabetes. J Clin Pharm Ther 2012;37(2):187–95.

21. Garvey W, Ryan D, Look M, et al. Two-year sustained weight loss and metabolic benefits with controlled-release phentermine/topiramate in obese and overweight adults (SEQUEL): a randomized, placebo-controlled, phase 3 extension study. Am J Clin Nutr 2012;95(2):297–308.

22. Farquhar C, Brown J, Marjoribanks J. Laparoscopic drilling by diathermy or laser for ovulation induction in anovulatory polycystic ovary syndrome. Cochrane Database Syst Rev 2012;(6):CD001122.

23. Use of clomiphene citrate in women. Fertil Steril 2006;86(5):187–93.

24. Dovey S, Sneeringer R, Penzias A. Clomiphene citrate and intrauterine insemination: analysis of more than 4100 cycles. Fertil Steril 2008;90(6):2281–6.

25. Imani B. A nomogram to predict the probability of live birth after clomiphene citrate induction of ovulation in normogonadotropic oligoamenorrheic infertility. Fertil Steril 2002;71(1):91–7.

26. Pritts EA, Yuen AK, Sharma S, et al. The use of high dose letrozole in ovulation induction and controlled ovarian hyperstimulation. ISRN Obstet Gynecol 2011; 2011:242864.

27. Barbieri RL. Metformin for the treatment of polycystic ovary syndrome. Obstet Gynecol 2003;101(4):785–93.

28. Haas DA, Carr BR, Attia GR. Effects of metformin on body mass index, menstrual cyclicity, and ovulation induction in women with polycystic ovary syndrome. Fertil Steril 2003;79(3):469–81.

29. Maciel GA, Soares Junior JM, Alves da Motta EL, et al. Nonobese women with polycystic ovary syndrome respond better than obese women to treatment with metformin. Fertil Steril 2004;81(2):355–60.

30. Nestler JE, Jakubowicz DJ. Decreases in ovarian cytochrome P450c17 alpha activity and serum free testosterone after reduction of insulin secretion in polycystic ovary syndrome. N Engl J Med 1996;335(9):617–23.

31. Niskanen L, Uusitupa M, Sarlund H, et al. The effects of weight loss on insulin sensitivity, skeletal muscle composition and capillary density in obese non-diabetic subjects. Int J Obes Relat Metab Disord 1996;20(2):154–60.

32. Blonde L, Dailey GE, Jabbour SA, et al. Gastrointestinal tolerability of extended-release metformin tablets compared to immediate-release metformin tablets: results of a retrospective cohort study. Curr Med Res Opin 2004;20(4): 565–72.

33. Glueck CJ, Goldenberg N, Pranikoff J, et al. Height, weight, and motor-social development during the first 18 months of life in 126 infants born to 109 mothers with polycystic ovary syndrome who conceived on and continued metformin through pregnancy. Hum Reprod 2004;19(6):1323–30.

34. Jakubowicz DJ, Iuorno MJ, Jakubowicz S, et al. Effects of metformin on early pregnancy loss in the polycystic ovary syndrome. J Clin Endocrinol Metab 2002;87(2):524–9.

35. Nestler JE, Jakubowicz DJ, Evans WS, et al. Effects of metformin on spontaneous and clomiphene-induced ovulation in the polycystic ovary syndrome. N Engl J Med 1998;338(26):1876–80.

36. Palomba S, Orio F Jr, Falbo A, et al. Prospective parallel randomized, double-blind, double-dummy controlled clinical trial comparing clomiphene citrate and metformin as the first-line treatment for ovulation induction in nonobese anovulatory women with polycystic ovary syndrome. J Clin Endocrinol Metab 2005;90(7):4068–74.

37. Legro RS, Barnhart HX, Schlaff WD, et al. Clomiphene, metformin, or both for infertility in the polycystic ovary syndrome. N Engl J Med 2007;356(6):551–66.

38. Siebert TI, Viola MI, Steyn DW, et al. Is metformin indicated as primary ovulation induction agent in women with PCOS? a systematic review and meta-analysis. Gynecol Obstet Invest 2012;73(4):304–13.

39. Morin-Papunen L, Rantala AS, Unkila-Kallio L, et al. Metformin Improves Pregnancy and Live-Birth Rates in Women with Polycystic Ovary Syndrome (PCOS): a multicenter, double-blind, placebo-controlled randomized trial. J Clin Endocrinol Metab 2012;97(5):1492–500.

40. Nezhat C, Nezhat F, Nezhat C. Nezhat's operative gynecologic laparoscopy and hysteroscopy. New York: Cambridge University Press; 2008.

41. Thessaloniki ESHRE/ASRM-Sponsored PCOS Consensus Workshop Group. Consensus on infertility treatment related to polycystic ovary syndrome. Fertil Steril 2008;89(3):505–22.

42. Amer SA, Li TC, Metwally M, et al. Randomized controlled trial comparing laparoscopic ovarian diathermy with clomiphene citrate as a first-line method of ovulation induction in women with polycystic ovary syndrome. Hum Reprod 2009;24(1):219–25.

43. Palomba S, Orio F Jr, Nardo LG, et al. Metformin administration versus laparoscopic ovarian diathermy in clomiphene citrate-resistant women with polycystic ovary syndrome: a prospective parallel randomized double-blind placebo-controlled trial. J Clin Endocrinol Metab 2004;89(10):4801–9.

44. Dokras A, Clifton S, Futterweit W, et al. Increased risk for abnormal depression scores in women with polycystic ovary syndrome: a systematic review and meta-analysis. Obstet Gynecol 2011;117(1):145–52.

45. Nandalike K, Agarwal C, Strauss T, et al. Sleep and cardiometabolic function in obese adolescent girls with polycystic ovary syndrome. pii: S1389–9457. Sleep Med 2012;(12):00285–7.

Evaluation and Treatment of Anovulatory and Unexplained Infertility

Anthony M. Propst, MD[a], G. Wright Bates Jr, MD[b],*

KEYWORDS

- Anovulatory disorders • Unexplained infertility • Polycystic ovarian syndrome
- Obesity

KEY POINTS

- A low-caloric diet and a structured exercise program should be recommended for obese anovulatory women.
- Clomiphene citrate is the initial treatment for most women with ovulatory dysfunction and unexplained infertility.
- Ovulation induction monitoring may be useful to document ovulation and for the timing of intercourse or intrauterine insemination.
- Letrozole is an option for women who have failed to ovulate or conceive as well as for those with thin endometrial lining or bothersome side effects using clomiphene citrate.
- Gonadotropins are second-line agents for anovulation and require close observation because of the high rates of multiple pregnancies.
- The role of laparoscopy in the evaluation and treatment of ovulatory disorders or unexplained infertility is unclear.

INFERTILITY AND OVULATORY DYSFUNCTION

With an average monthly fecundity rate of only 20%, human beings are not fertile compared with other mammals.[1] Overall, 10% to 15% of couples have difficulties conceiving, or conceiving the number of children they want, and many will seek specialist fertility care at least once during their reproductive lifetime. Infertility is

Dr Propst has nothing to disclose. Dr Propst is a Colonel in the United States Air Force Medical Corps. The opinions and conclusions in this article are those of the author and are not intended to represent the official position of the Department of Defense, United States Air Force, or any other government agency.

a Department of Obstetrics and Gynecology, Uniformed Services University of the Health Sciences, 4301 Jones Bridge Road, Bethesda, MD 20814, USA; b Department of Obstetrics and Gynecology, University of Alabama School of Medicine, 10390 Women and Infants Center, 1700 6th Avenue South, Birmingham, AL, USA
* Corresponding author.
E-mail address: wbates@uab.edu

Obstet Gynecol Clin N Am 39 (2012) 507–519
http://dx.doi.org/10.1016/J.ogc.2012.09.008
0889-8545/12/$ – see front matter © 2012 Elsevier Inc. All rights reserved.

obgyn.theclinics.com

a disease defined as the failure to conceive after 12 months of regular unprotected intercourse in a reproductive-aged couple. Beginning the fertility evaluation prior to one year of infertility is warranted when the woman has known or suspected anovulation or tubal factor, is older than 35 years, or if her partner has a suspected male factor.[2] Infertility affects a large number of couples. National surveys indicate that 11% of nulliparous married women younger than 29 years have nonvoluntary infertility and that rate increases to 27% of nulliparous married women aged 40 to 44 years.[3]

Ovulatory dysfunction is one of the major causes of infertility, affecting 25% of couples with infertility.[4] The World Health Organization (WHO) has classified anovulation into 3 categories.[5]

1. WHO I is anovulation with low gonadotropin levels, sometimes referred to as hypogonadotropic hypogonadism. Women with this form of anovulation have low levels of endogenous estrogen, do not develop an adequate endometrial lining, and will usually not bleed when given a progestin challenge to induce progestin withdrawal bleeding. Clinically, these women will often have a body mass index less than 20 and are involved in high-intensity exercise or have high stress levels. In addition, they usually do not respond to oral ovulation induction medications because of hypothalamic-pituitary dysfunction and will usually need injectable gonadotropins that directly stimulate the ovarian follicles to ovulate.
2. WHO II is anovulation with normal levels of gonadotropins. Women with this type of anovulation make endogenous estrogen and will usually respond with menstrual bleeding when given a progestin challenge. Polycystic ovarian syndrome (PCOS) is an example of this type of ovulatory disorder. Clinically, these women usually have a functioning hypothalamus and pituitary system and generally respond to oral ovulation induction medications.
3. WHO III is anovulation with elevated gonadotropins. Women of reproductive age who have elevated gonadotropins are usually a result of premature ovarian failure, either caused by unknown causes or caused by ovarian damage from chemotherapy, radiation, or surgery. Clinically, these women have limited ovarian follicles that are not responding to high endogenous follicle-stimulating hormone (FSH) stimulation. Similarly, they do not respond to additional ovarian stimulation through fertility medications and usually require third-party reproduction, such as an egg donor, to conceive.

POLYCYSTIC OVARIAN SYNDROME

Most women with anovulatory infertility have PCOS, and most women with PCOS are overweight or obese. This combination requires careful attention to the morbidities associated with obesity and the need for lifestyle intervention with exercise and dietary changes to achieve weight loss. PCOS prevalence in the population and impact on reproduction as well as overall health warrants special consideration. PCOS is covered in depth in the article by Bates and Propst elsewhere in this issue.

UNEXPLAINED INFERTILITY

Approximately 25% of couples will have no identifiable cause for their subfertility following a routine evaluation.[6] The diagnosis of unexplained infertility requires a normal semen analysis with evidence of tubal patency and ovulation. As one would surmise, the absences of an abnormal finding does not preclude the presence of an obstacle to normal reproduction (**Table 1**). However, exhaustive testing or pursuit of potential causes of infertility, in most cases, will not increase the efficacy of treatment

Table 1	
Assessment of endocrine function in infertility patients	
Endocrine System Screened	**Laboratory Test**
Thyroid	Thyroid stimulating hormone
Pituitary	Prolactin
Androgen excess	Total and free testosterone, DHEA-S
Congenital adrenal hyperplasia	17-OH progesterone
Cushing syndrome	24-h urine cortisol or overnight dexamethasone suppression test

Abbreviations: DHEA-S, Dehydroepiandrosterone Sulfate; 17-OH, 17-hydroxyprogesterone.
   Data from Kamath MS, Bhattacharya S. Demographics of infertility and management of unexplained infertility. Best Pract Res Clin Obstet Gynaecol 2012 Aug 27. [Epub ahead of print].

or the potential for a successful delivery. Likewise, treatment aimed at achieving a successful pregnancy in women with unexplained infertility is by definition empiric, and much controversy surrounds the risk versus benefit of ovulation induction in this population. The clinician must weigh the potential benefit based on inconclusive data with the known risk of multiple gestations and other possible negative sequelae of supraphysiologic estrogen levels.

FERTILE WINDOW

There are a limited number of days in a menstrual cycle when a woman is fertile. In a landmark study that defined the fertility window, investigators looked at the timing of intercourse in relation to ovulation for 221 couples and evaluated subsequent pregnancy rates.[7] This study found that the fertile window begins 5 days before ovulation and ends on the day of ovulation. The highest likelihood of becoming pregnant is from 2 days before ovulation until the day of ovulation, with the pregnancy likelihood of approximately 35% on those 3 days. In a European study of 770 couples using natural family planning methods of contraception, 650 couples had intercourse at least once during the preovulatory period they were supposed to be abstaining, resulting in 433 pregnancies.[8] This study also found that the fertile window begins 5 days before ovulation and ends at ovulation, with the peak fecundity occurring with intercourse 2 days before ovulation. Women are most fertile the 2 days before ovulation and should be instructed to time intercourse during this period so that sperm are present in the genital tract before the follicle ovulates and releases the oocyte.

OVULATION INDUCTION MONITORING

When using medications for ovulation induction, it is imperative to document ovulation or lack thereof. Knowing whether or not ovulation has occurred allows not only for proper timing of intercourse or intrauterine insemination (IUI) but also helps define the method of therapy for subsequent cycles in the event ovulation does not occur. Several methods exist to access ovulation ranging from minimal to invasive testing.

1. The presence of regular menses and moliminal symptoms before menses is a sign that the woman is ovulatory. The luteal phase following ovulation to menses is typically 14 days, regardless of the length of time between menses. Ovulation typically occurs on day 10 of a 24-day menstrual cycle, day 14 of a 28-day menstrual cycle, and day 21 of a 35-day menstrual cycle.

2. Basal body temperature measurements are an inexpensive method of detecting ovulation.[9] The body temperature will increase slightly after ovulation in response to an increase in endogenous progesterone. The cumbersome nature of monitoring daily temperatures first thing in the morning and because the temperature increase will occur only after ovulation and the fertility window is closed make charting basal body temperature less useful than other ovulation detection methods.

3. Urine luteinizing hormone (LH) detection kits detect the endogenous LH surge that occurs 36 to 48 hours before ovulation.[10] This method seems to be an easy and reliable method that patients are compliant with. Testing should begin 4 days before expected ovulation, based on the cycle length. Digital and nondigital ovulation predictor kits are available. The digital kits are more expensive but easier to interpret and are preferred by volunteers over the nondigital kits.[11] Once LH has been detected in the urine, patients should be instructed to have intercourse that day and the following day or scheduled for an IUI. Detection of ovulation and proper timing of intercourse doubled the chances of conception (odds ratio 1.89) in a cohort of women with no known obstacles to pregnancy.[12] This finding raises the possibility that a subset of unexplained infertility may be caused by poorly timed intercourse.

4. Luteal serum progesterone levels can also be measured to confirm that ovulation has occurred. When ovulation has occurred, the midluteal phase serum progesterone is greater than 3 ng/mL and preferably greater than 10 ng/mL. Serum progesterone should be measured approximately 1 week after expected ovulation. This practice will document ovulation but provides no guidance in the timing of intercourse or IUI.[13]

5. For patients that have difficulty detecting ovulation by ovulation predictor kits, ovarian follicular development can be monitored by ultrasound. When the lead follicle is 20 mm or more, ovulation can be induced with an injection of human chorionic gonadotropin (hCG). A recent retrospective study found a higher pregnancy rate when the lead follicle was 23 to 28 mm when given hCG.[14] Intercourse or an IUI can be timed for 12 to 36 hours following the hCG injection. Alternatively, the IUI can be scheduled after detecting ovulation using an LH detection kit. However, using LH testing results in higher rates of canceled cycles because of a false-negative rate of approximately 15% with LH testing.[15]

MEDICAL AND SURGICAL TREATMENT OPTIONS
Clomiphene Citrate

A variety of medications can be used to induce ovulation in women with ovulatory dysfunction. The most common initial ovulation induction medication is clomiphene citrate (CC), which can be combined with timed intercourse or IUI. CC is a nonsteroidal triphenylethylene derivative that has both estrogen agonist and antagonist properties.[9] CC was approved for clinical use in 1967 and predominately acts as an estrogen antagonist. CC binds to the estrogen receptors primarily in the hypothalamus. The prolonged binding of CC to the estrogen receptors interrupts the negative feedback of the increasing estrogen level and results in continued production of FSH, which stimulates follicular growth and maturation.[9] It is indicated for use in anovulatory women with normal thyroid and prolactin and who produce endogenous estrogen. It is also indicated for the empiric treatment of women with unexplained infertility when it is most effective when combined with IUI.[9]

CC is administered orally, beginning 3 to 5 days after the onset of a spontaneous or progestin-induced menses.[9] Contrary to traditional practice, a recent study suggested that women with anovulatory women with PCOS who began CC without first having a progestin withdrawal had significantly higher conception and live birth rates than women who took a progestin to induce menses before starting CC.[16] Treatment typically begins with a single 50-mg tablet daily for 5 days. Ovulation usually occurs within 5 to 10 days after the last dose of CC. It is important to confirm ovulation in patients that are using CC and to continue with the lowest dose that achieves ovulation. There is no benefit to increasing the dose if patients ovulate but do not get pregnant during that cycle. If patients remain anovulatory, the dose should be increased. Most patients that will ovulate on CC will ovulate at the 100-mg dose or less, with decreasing rates of ovulation at higher doses for patients resistant at the 100-mg dose. The United States Food and Drug Administration's maximum recommended dose is 100 mg/d for 5 days; however, some physicians will continue to increase the dose in 50-mg increments up to 250 mg until ovulation is achieved.[9] Some CC-resistant women who fail to ovulate with a 5-day regimen of 250 mg/d may respond to an 8-day course of the same dose.[17]

The use of CC in anovulatory women results in ovulation rates of approximately 75% and overall pregnancy rates of 50% to 70% of those who ovulate and continue the medication for up to 12 cycles.[18,19] Cycle fecundity is approximately 15% in anovulatory women who ovulate in response to CC. Most conceptions occur within the first 6 ovulatory cycles. Most women (88%) who conceive with the assistance of CC do so at doses of 150 mg or less and 52% conceive at doses of 50 mg.[19] If ovulation has not occurred at 100-mg or 150-mg doses, complimentary or alternative medications for ovulation induction should be implemented, which is discussed later.

Similar to ovulatory women, the fecundity rate for women using CC decreases with age. In a large retrospective analysis of 4000 CC cycles with IUI of anovulation and unexplained infertility, the per-cycle fecundity rates were 10% for women younger than 35 years but 4% or less for women aged 41 years or older.[20]

Empiric treatment with CC for couples with unexplained infertility is a first-line therapy. CC or IUI as individual treatments do not improve the baseline chance of conception each month (fecundity) compared with historical controls, but the combination of CC with IUI can double the monthly fecundity rate.[21]

The incidence of multiple gestations with the use of CC is approximately 8% and most of these are twins. Triplet or higher-order multiple births are rare but can occur.[9] The most common side effect is vasomotor symptoms, which occur in approximately 10% of women taking CC. Less common side effects include mood swings, breast tenderness, headaches, and nausea. Visual disturbances occur in less than 2% but occasionally can be permanent, and CC use should be stopped in patients who have them.

There is not an increase of congenital anomalies or birth defects in the children conceived by women taking CC. Although some retrospective studies have reported an increased risk of ovarian cancer, overall there does not seem to be an increase in the incidence of ovarian or breast cancer in infertile women who have taken CC.[22,23]

Letrozole

Letrozole is an aromatase inhibitor that blocks the conversion of androgens to estrogens. Letrozole is indicated for the treatment of postmenopausal women with hormone-receptor-positive or unknown breast cancer. However, it is increasingly being used off label for ovulation induction. Letrozole's mechanism of action for ovulation induction is thought to be the release of the hypothalamus and the pituitary from the negative feedback of estrogen (**Fig. 1**).[24] With a lower estradiol level, there is less negative feedback on the hypothalamus and pituitary and the levels of GnRH and,

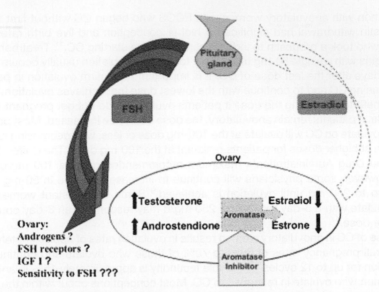

Fig. 1. Hypothalamic Pituitary Ovarian Axis and Aromatase Inhibition. IGF, Insulin like Growth Factor. (*From* Holzer H, Casper R, Tulandi T. A new era in ovulation induction. Fertil Steril 2006;85(2):277–84; with permission.)

therefore, FSH is increased, which leads to further stimulation of follicular development. Letrozole can be used to stimulate ovulation in women who do not respond to CC or in women that have side effects with CC, such as uncomfortable vasomotor symptoms, visual changes, or headaches.[25] These side effects are rare in patients using letrozole for ovulation induction. Some patients will have a thin endometrium (less than 7 mm) when taking CC. The proliferation of the endometrium is stimulated by estrogen. Because CC acts as an estrogen antagonist, in some women the endometrial lining is thin, which may reduce implantation. Letrozole does not have the same antiestrogen effect on the endometrium.[26,27] Letrozole can be used in combination of timed intercourse or IUI.

Letrozole is typically prescribed at a starting dose of 2.5 to 5.0 mg and can be increased by increments of 2.5 mg.[28] The highest commonly used dose is 7.5 mg. It is given for 5 consecutive days like CC and can be started as early as day 3 of the cycle. A recent publication reported using letrozole at higher doses, up to 12.5 mg/d, with high rates of ovulation among patients who did not respond to lower doses.[29]

The first report of letrozole being used as an ovulation induction medication was published in 2001 and looked at 12 women who had failed to ovulate with CC treatment and an additional 10 women who ovulated on CC but who had an endometrial thickness of 5 mm or less.[26] Letrozole 2.5 mg was given for 5 days (day 3 to 7). The rate of ovulation increased from 44% while taking CC to 75% with letrozole. The endometrial thickness went from 5 mm or less with CC to a mean endometrial thickness of 8 mm with letrozole.

Several studies have looked at letrozole versus CC as a first-line therapy in women with anovulatory infertility (**Table 2**).[28] Begum and colleagues[27] looked at the rate of ovulation, endometrial thickness, and pregnancy rates between 64 women who failed to ovulate when taking CC 100 mg. These women were randomly assigned to either CC 150 mg or letrozole 7.5 mg for 5 days. This study showed higher rates of ovulation (62.5% vs 37.5%) endometrial thickness, and overall pregnancy rate (40.6% vs 18.8%) in to the letrozole group compared with the CC group.

Table 2
RCTs comparing letrozole versus clomiphene as first line for anovulatory women

S. No.	Authors	Study Design	Treatment Arms	Numbers Cycles	Endometrial Thickness (mm)	Ovulation Rates (%)	Pregnancy Rates (%)
1	Atay et al,[30] Turkey, 2006	RCT	Letrozole 2.5 mg vs clomiphene 100 mg	51 vs 55	8.4 ± 1.8 vs 5.2 ± 1.2	82.4 vs 63.6	21.6 vs 9.1
2	Bayar et al,[10] Turkey, 2006	RCT	Letrozole 2.5 mg vs clomiphene 100 mg	99 vs 95	8[a] vs 8[a]	65.7 vs 74.7	9.1 vs 7.4
3	Badawy et al,[31] Egypt, 2009	RCT	Letrozole 5 mg vs clomiphene 100 mg	540 vs 523	8.1 ± 0.2 vs 9.2 ± 0.7	67.5 vs 70.9	15.1 vs 17.9

Abbreviation: RCT, randomized controlled trial.
[a] Values represent median.
Data from Kamath MS, George K. Letrozole or clomiphene citrate as first line for anovulatory infertility: a debate. Reprod Biol Endocrinol 2011;9:86.

Atay and colleagues[30] performed a randomized controlled trial (RCT) that evaluated 106 women with PCOS to receive either letrozole (2.5 mg) or CC (100 mg) for 5 days. The ovulation rates (82.4% vs 63.6%) and clinical pregnancy rates (21.6% vs 9.1%) were significantly higher in the letrozole group. However, in the largest RCT, involving more than 400 women and 1000 cycles, Badawy and colleagues[31] compared letrozole versus CC for women with PCOS and found similar ovulation (67.5% vs 70.9%) and pregnancy rates (15.1% vs 17.9%). The investigators concluded that there was no benefit for letrozole over CC, especially because letrozole is more expensive than CC.

A review of clinicaltrials.gov shows that several trials are underway that evaluate CC versus letrozole, including 2 by the National Institutes of Child Health and Human Development's The Reproductive Medicine Network. The first, Pregnancy in Polycystic Ovarian Syndrome II, is comparing letrozole versus CC for women with PCOS, whereas the Assessment of Multiple Intrauterine Gestations from Ovarian Stimulation trial is assessing the risk and benefit of superovulation with letrozole, CC, or gonadotropins in women with unexplained infertility.

One advantage of letrozole is that it has a lower incidence of multiple pregnancies when compared with CC or gonadotropins.[32] Several years ago, there was some concern raised about higher rates of birth defects in women conceived after taking letrozole. An abstract presentation at the American Society for Reproductive Medicine in 2005 suggested an increased risk of congenital malformation compared with a low-risk obstetric control group. The manufacturer of letrozole (Novartis) subsequently sent a warning letter to doctors that letrozole was not to be used as an ovulation induction medication. However, a succeeding Canadian study of more than 900 infants that compared the birth defects of infants born to mothers taking letrozole versus CC found similar rates of defects in the letrozole infants and the CC infants (2.4% vs 4.8%).[33] Patients should be informed that letrozole is being prescribed off label so they can make an informed decision and are not concerned when they read the package instructions.

Gonadotropins

The administration of exogenous FSH or human menopausal gonadotropin is considered the second line of therapy for ovulation induction for patients who do not respond to oral therapy or have been unsuccessful in achieving a pregnancy.[34] Gonadotropins are the first line of treatment of ovulation induction in the WHO I category of hypogonadotropic hypogonadism because patients are not producing adequate levels of FSH and LH and do not respond to oral medications, such as CC or Letrozole.[5]

When starting gonadotropins, patients must understand the expense of the medications as well as the commitment required in monitoring the effects of the medication. Close monitoring of serum estradiol levels and follicular number and growth by an experienced physician is mandatory to minimize the risks of high-order multiple pregnancies (HOMP). The key is to start with lower dosages of medication, 50 to 100 IU daily. Clinical judgment is necessary in dosing the medication and adjusting the dose throughout the cycle according to estradiol levels and follicular growth.

There are significant risks of twins (11%) and high-order multiples (3.0%–4.1%) when using gonadotropins.[35] HOMP are positively related to the use of high doses of gonadotropin, higher number of 7- to 10-mm preovulatory follicles, and higher estradiol.[36] HOMP are also more common in younger patients. For women aged younger than 32 years, HOMP was 6% for 3 to 6 follicles and 20% for 7 or more follicles. For women aged 32 to 37 years, HOMP was 5% for 3 to 6 follicles and 12% for 7 or more follicles. HOMP are also most likely to occur in the first gonadotropin treatment cycle and were rare after the second treatment cycle.[37]

Strategies successful in reducing HOMP include using CC earlier in the cycle before starting gonadotropins, using low gonadotropin doses, cancellation for more than 3 follicles that are more than 10 to 15 mm. By using a conservative strategy, 5% to 20% of cycles may be canceled but HOMP rates can be less than 2% and pregnancy rates can average 10% to 20% per cycle.[36]

Metformin

Metformin is an antihyperglycemic that is widely used off label as an adjunct to ovulation induction or superovulation. The net effect of lowering serum glucose in women who are anovulatory is a reduction of androgens and potential resumptions in ovulation.[38] Although numerous case series and cohort studies have demonstrated a favorable impact on pregnancy rates following ovulation induction, randomized trials have yielded mixed results.[39–41] Metformin has not been shown to increase the chances of a live birth in women with unexplained infertility. The role of metformin in the treatment of PCOS and ovulation induction is examined at length in the article by Bates and Propst elsewhere in this issue.

Glucocorticoids and Clomiphene Citrate

In cases of CC resistance in the setting of normal and elevated dehydroepiandrosterone, daily dexamethasone (0.5–2.0 mg) or prednisone (5 mg) during the follicular phase have been used adjunctively with CC. The combination of glucocorticoids and CC has been shown to significantly increase the rate of ovulation and pregnancy when compared with CC alone in randomized trials.[42–44]

Oral Contraceptives and Clomiphene Citrate

Two months of oral contraceptive pill treatment before ovulation induction with CC may improve the observed rate of ovulation and pregnancy.[45] Treatment with Oral Contraceptive Pills (OCPs) is associated with lower levels of testosterone and androstenedione, which probably accounts for the improved ovarian response to CC.

Timed Intercourse Versus IUI

The decision to proceed with timed intercourse or IUI has to do with the quality of the partner's semen; the presence of a cervical factor, such as cervical stenosis; and the previous treatment history of the patient. Semen analyses can vary based on illness, stress, and recent ejaculations. A long abstinence interval increases the sperm count but decreases the percent motile and IUI pregnancy rates.[46] Higher pregnancy rates are seen in daily or every-other-day intercourse versus once weekly because the percentage of normal sperm seems to correlate with the frequency of ejaculations.[10]

If an abnormal semen analysis is obtained, it is best to repeat it 6 to 8 weeks later. After 3 cycles of ovulation and timed intercourse, IUI should be recommended. However, if the total motile sperm count is less than 10 million, in vitro fertilization or intracytoplasmic sperm injection is the most cost-effective treatment.[47]

For women with anovulation and a partner with a normal semen analysis, timed intercourse after ovulation induction is the authors' recommended first-line treatment. For couples with unexplained infertility, IUI will improve success rates with both CC and gonadotropins compared with timed intercourse or intracervical insemination.[21,48]

Laparoscopy

Laparoscopy has become the gold standard for the diagnosis and surgical treatment of pelvic pathology. However, its role in the evaluation and treatment of infertility has become less clear with the advent and success of assisted reproductive technologies

(ART). Some investigators argue that the diagnosis of unexplained infertility cannot be made without a surgical or laparoscopy confirmation of normal pelvic anatomy. A recent trial of diagnostic laparoscopy found pelvic pathology in 83% of women with a normal routine fertility evaluation who failed to conceive following 3 months of ovulation induction. The investigators also suggested that surgical intervention increased the chances of pregnancy.[49] Others have argued that even in the presence of tubal occlusion due to prior tubal ligation, adhesions and/or endometriosis, surgical intervention is inferior to ART.[50]

One possible exception to the purported demise of reproduction surgery can be found in laparoscopic ovarian drilling (LOD). This use of thermal energy to damage the ovarian cortex and reduce production of androgen has been recommended as the second-line therapy for patients with PCOS who are resistant to ovulation induction.[34] Although LOD has a significantly lower risk of multiple pregnancies, the live birth rate is also lower when compared with ovulation induction agents.[51] Nonetheless, laparoscopy and LOD may play a role in properly selecting women for whom advanced ovulation induction is not practical or available or for those who wish to avoid the risk of multiple gestations and/or the use of gonadotropins.

SUMMARY RECOMMENDATIONS

- A low-caloric diet and a structured exercise program should be recommended for obese anovulatory women. These lifestyle changes can result in weight loss and spontaneous ovulation.
- CC is the initial treatment for most women with ovulatory dysfunction and unexplained infertility. CC should be started at 50 mg for 5 days of the cycle, starting between the third and fifth day of the cycle. The dose can be increased by 50 mg if patients do not ovulate but should not be increased if ovulation is occurring.
- Once ovulation induction methods are prescribed, some type of ovulation induction monitoring should be performed and ovulation should be documented.
- Letrozole is an option for women who have failed to ovulate using CC. It is typically started at a dosage of 2.5 to 5.0 mg for 5 days of the cycle, starting between the third and fifth day of the cycle. Letrozole is also beneficial when patients have an endometrial lining of 6 mm or less on CC or patients have bothersome side effects on CC.
- Gonadotropins are second-line agents for anovulation. They should be used with caution because of the high rates of multiple pregnancies and require close observation of the developing follicular size and number.
- Laparoscopic ovarian diathermy may play a limited role as a second-line intervention for patients with PCOS. Laparoscopy's role in the evaluation of unexplained infertility is controversial.

REFERENCES

1. Evers JL. Female subfertility. Lancet 2002;360(9327):151–9.
2. Practice Committee of the American Society for Reproductive Medicine. Definitions of infertility and recurrent pregnancy loss. Fertil Steril 2008;89(6):1603.
3. Chandra A, et al. Fertility, family planning, and reproductive health of U.S. women: data from the 2002 national survey of family growth. Vital Health Stat 23 2005;(25):1–160.
4. ACOG Committee on Practice Bulletins-Gynecology. ACOG practice bulletin. Clinical management guidelines for obstetrician-gynecologists number 34, February 2002. Management of infertility caused by ovulatory dysfunction.

American College of Obstetricians and Gynecologists. Obstet Gynecol 2002; 99(2):347–58.

5. Agents stimulating gonadal function in the human. Report of a WHO scientific group. World Health Organ Tech Rep Ser 1973;514:1–30.

6. Kamath MS, Bhattacharya S. Demographics of infertility and management of unexplained infertility. Best Pract Res Clin Obstet Gynaecol 2012. [Epub ahead of print].

7. Wilcox AJ, Weinberg CR, Baird DD. Timing of sexual intercourse in relation to ovulation. Effects on the probability of conception, survival of the pregnancy, and sex of the baby. N Engl J Med 1995;333(23):1517–21.

8. Dunson DB, Colombo B, Baird DD. Changes with age in the level and duration of fertility in the menstrual cycle. Hum Reprod 2002;17(5):1399–403.

9. Practice Committee of the American Society for Reproductive Medicine. Use of clomiphene citrate in women. Fertil Steril 2006;86(5 Suppl 1):S187–93.

10. Practice Committee of American Society for Reproductive Medicine in collaboration with Society for Reproductive Endocrinology and Infertility. Optimizing natural fertility. Fertil Steril 2008;90(Suppl 5):S1–6.

11. Tomlinson C, Marshall J, Ellis JE. Comparison of accuracy and certainty of results of six home pregnancy tests available over-the-counter. Curr Med Res Opin 2008; 24(6):1645–9.

12. Robinson J, Wakelin M, Ellis J. Increased pregnancy rate with use of the Clearblue Easy fertility monitor. Fertil Steril 2007;2:329–34.

13. Wathen NC, et al. Interpretation of single progesterone measurement in diagnosis of anovulation and defective luteal phase: observations on analysis of the normal range. Br Med J (Clin Res Ed) 1984;288(6410):7–9.

14. Palatnik A, et al. What is the optimal follicular size before triggering ovulation in intrauterine insemination cycles with clomiphene citrate or letrozole? An analysis of 988 cycles. Fertil Steril 2012;97(5):1089–94.e1–3.

15. Lewis V, et al. Clomiphene citrate monitoring for intrauterine insemination timing: a randomized trial. Fertil Steril 2006;85(2):401–6.

16. Diamond MP, et al. Endometrial shedding effect on conception and live birth in women with polycystic ovary syndrome. Obstet Gynecol 2012;119(5):902–8.

17. Lobo RA, et al. An extended regimen of clomiphene citrate in women unresponsive to standard therapy. Fertil Steril 1982;37(6):762–6.

18. Imani B, et al. Predictors of chances to conceive in ovulatory patients during clomiphene citrate induction of ovulation in normogonadotropic oligoamenorrheic infertility. J Clin Endocrinol Metab 1999;84(5):1617–22.

19. Imani B, et al. A nomogram to predict the probability of live birth after clomiphene citrate induction of ovulation in normogonadotropic oligoamenorrheic infertility. Fertil Steril 2002;77(1):91–7.

20. Dovey S, Sneeringer RM, Penzias AS. Clomiphene citrate and intrauterine insemination: analysis of more than 4100 cycles. Fertil Steril 2008;90(6):2281–6.

21. Guzick DS, et al. Efficacy of treatment for unexplained infertility. Fertil Steril 1998; 70(2):207–13.

22. Zreik TG, et al. Fertility drugs and risk of ovarian cancer: dispelling the myth. Curr Opin Obstet Gynecol 2008;20(3):313–9.

23. Sanner K, et al. Ovarian epithelial neoplasia after hormonal infertility treatment: long-term follow-up of a historical cohort in Sweden. Fertil Steril 2009;91(4): 1152–8.

24. Holzer H, Casper R, Tulandi T. A new era in ovulation induction. Fertil Steril 2006; 85(2):277–84.

25. Nahid L, Sirous K. Comparison of the effects of letrozole and clomiphene citrate for ovulation induction in infertile women with polycystic ovary syndrome. Minerva Ginecol 2012;64(3):253–8.
26. Mitwally MF, Casper RF. Use of an aromatase inhibitor for induction of ovulation in patients with an inadequate response to clomiphene citrate. Fertil Steril 2001; 75(2):305–9.
27. Begum MR, et al. Comparison of efficacy of aromatase inhibitor and clomiphene citrate in induction of ovulation in polycystic ovarian syndrome. Fertil Steril 2009; 92(3):853–7.
28. Kamath MS, George K. Letrozole or clomiphene citrate as first line for anovulatory infertility: a debate. Reprod Biol Endocrinol 2011;9:86.
29. Pritts EA, et al. The use of high dose letrozole in ovulation induction and controlled ovarian hyperstimulation. ISRN Obstet Gynecol 2011;2011:242864.
30. Atay V, et al. Comparison of letrozole and clomiphene citrate in women with polycystic ovaries undergoing ovarian stimulation. J Int Med Res 2006;34(1): 73–6.
31. Badawy A, Abdel Aal I, Abulatta M. Clomiphene citrate or letrozole for ovulation induction in women with polycystic ovarian syndrome: a prospective randomized trial. Fertil Steril 2009;92(3):849–52.
32. Mitwally MF, Biljan MM, Casper RF. Pregnancy outcome after the use of an aromatase inhibitor for ovarian stimulation. Am J Obstet Gynecol 2005;192(2):381–6.
33. Tulandi T, et al. Congenital malformations among 911 newborns conceived after infertility treatment with letrozole or clomiphene citrate. Fertil Steril 2006;85(6): 1761–5.
34. Thessaloniki ESHRE/ASRM-Sponsored PCOS Consensus Workshop Group. Consensus on infertility treatment related to polycystic ovary syndrome. Fertil Steril 2008;89(3):505–22.
35. Kaplan PF, et al. Assessing the risk of multiple gestation in gonadotropin intrauterine insemination cycles. Am J Obstet Gynecol 2002;186(6):1244–7 [discussion: 1247–9].
36. Dickey RP. Strategies to reduce multiple pregnancies due to ovulation stimulation. Fertil Steril 2009;91(1):1–17.
37. Dickey RP, et al. Risk factors for high-order multiple pregnancy and multiple birth after controlled ovarian hyperstimulation: results of 4,062 intrauterine insemination cycles. Fertil Steril 2005;83(3):671–83.
38. Barbieri RL. Metformin for the treatment of polycystic ovary syndrome. Obstet Gynecol 2003;101(4):9.
39. Legro RS, et al. Clomiphene, metformin, or both for infertility in the polycystic ovary syndrome. N Engl J Med 2007;356(6):551–66.
40. Siebert T, et al. Is metformin indicated as primary ovulation induction agent in women with PCOS? A systematic review and meta-analysis. Gynecol Obstet Invest 2012;73(4):10.
41. Morin-Papunen L, et al. Metformin improves pregnancy and live-birth rates in women with polycystic ovary syndrome (PCOS): a multicenter, double-blind, placebo-controlled randomized trial. J Clin Endocrinol Metab 2012;97(5): 1492–500.
42. Daly DC, et al. A randomized study of dexamethasone in ovulation induction with clomiphene citrate. Fertil Steril 1984;41(6):844–8.
43. Isaacs JD Jr, Lincoln SR, Cowan BD. Extended clomiphene citrate (CC) and prednisone for the treatment of chronic anovulation resistant to CC alone. Fertil Steril 1997;67(4):641–3.

44. Elnashar A, et al. Clomiphene citrate and dexamethasone in treatment of clomiphene citrate-resistant polycystic ovary syndrome: a prospective placebo-controlled study. Hum Reprod 2006;21(7):1805–8.

45. Branigan EF, Estes MA. A randomized clinical trial of treatment of clomiphene citrate-resistant anovulation with the use of oral contraceptive pill suppression and repeat clomiphene citrate treatment. Am J Obstet Gynecol 2003;188(6): 1424–8 [discussion: 1429–30].

46. Jurema MW, et al. Effect of ejaculatory abstinence period on the pregnancy rate after intrauterine insemination. Fertil Steril 2005;84(3):678–81.

47. Van Voorhis BJ, et al. Effect of the total motile sperm count on the efficacy and cost-effectiveness of intrauterine insemination and in vitro fertilization. Fertil Steril 2001;75(4):661–8.

48. Guzick DS, et al. Efficacy of superovulation and intrauterine insemination in the treatment of infertility. National cooperative reproductive medicine network. N Engl J Med 1999;340(3):177–83.

49. Bonneau C, et al. Use of laparoscopy in unexplained infertility. Eur J Obstet Gynecol Reprod Biol 2012;163(1):57–61.

50. Feinberg E, Levens E, DeCherney A. Infertility surgery is dead: only the obituary remains? Fertil Steril 2008;89(1):232–6.

51. Farquhar C, Brown J, Marjoribanks J. Laparoscopic drilling by diathermy or laser for ovulation induction in anovulatory polycystic ovary syndrome. Cochrane Database Syst Rev 2012;6:CD001122.

The Impact and Management of Fibroids for Fertility

An Evidence-Based Approach

Xiaoxiao Catherine Guo, BS, James H. Segars, MD*

KEYWORDS

- Leiomyoma • Infertility • Assisted reproductive technology (ART) • Myomectomy
- Hysteroscopy • Minimally invasive gynecologic surgeries
- Magnetic resonance–guided focused ultrasound (MRgFUS)
- Uterine artery embolization (UAE)

KEY POINTS

- When selecting a treatment plan for symptomatic uterine fibroids, the fibroid location, size, and number will often dictate the proper intervention.
- Myomectomy is usually the best option for women desiring future fertility.
- Currently available medical therapies for uterine fibroids reduce symptoms, but are limited and most are confined to short-term use.
- Initial fertility studies on magnetic resonance–guided focused ultrasound and uterine artery embolization are encouraging, but randomized controlled trials need to be done. At this time, uterine artery embolization is not recommended for women desiring to become pregnant.
- Additional options for treating symptomatic uterine fibroids, including nonsurgical and preventative medical therapies, are still needed.

Uterine fibroids, or leiomyoma, are benign tumors of the uterus that may cause severe pain, bleeding, and infertility.[1] Fibroids affect a woman's quality of life, as well as her fertility and obstetric outcomes. Fibroids affect approximately 35% to 77% of reproductive-age women,[2–4] although the real prevalence is much higher because many fibroids may be asymptomatic. Nearing age 50, this likelihood may increase to 70% to 80% depending on the patient's ethnicity.[3] Of particular note, Peddada and colleagues[5] found that fibroid growth rates declined for white women older

Disclosure: The authors report no conflict of interest.

Reprint Requests: James H. Segars, MD; Xiaoxiao Catherine Guo, BS.

Program in Reproductive and Adult Endocrinology, *Eunice Kennedy Shriver* National Institute of Child Health and Human Development, National Institutes of Health, 10 Center Drive, Building 10 CRC 1-3140, MSC 1109, Bethesda, MD 20892-1109, USA

* Corresponding author.

E-mail address: segarsj@mail.nih.gov

Obstet Gynecol Clin N Am 39 (2012) 521–533

http://dx.doi.org/10.1016/j.ogc.2012.09.005

0889-8545/12/$ – see front matter Published by Elsevier Inc.

obgyn.theclinics.com

than 35 years but did not decline for black women of the same age. Fibroids are a public health concern and have been estimated to cost the US health care system up to $34.4 billion per year.[6]

In this review, we examine the medical and surgical therapies that women and their providers may choose to treat uterine fibroids, paying particular attention to pregnancy rates and obstetric outcomes. When selecting a treatment, individual patient preferences should be taken into account, such as desire for future childbearing. The fibroid location, size, and number are essential considerations.

Aside from traditional surgical therapies such as hysterectomy and myomectomy, minimally invasive gynecologic surgeries, uterine artery embolization (UAE), and magnetic resonance–guided focused ultrasound (MRgFUS) are increasing in popularity. The preliminary data using these newer therapies are encouraging. However, patients should be counseled that any uterus-sparing technique has the potential for fibroid recurrence.

FIBROIDS AND INFERTILITY

Fibroids are present in 5% to 10% of infertile patients and may be the sole cause of infertility in 1% to 2.4%.[7,8] Fibroids may cause infertility by obstructing the fallopian tubes and impairing gamete transport. It is now clear that the critical factor may be distortion of the endometrial cavity, causing abnormal endometrial receptivity, hormonal milieu, and altered endometrial development[9,10] (see later). However, the issue of whether fibroids can be the sole cause of infertility has been poorly understood.[7] This is because of the lack of prospective, randomized, and controlled studies separating out other infertility factors.[8] A randomized and prospective study evaluating spontaneous conception in infertile women with and without fibroids was conducted by Bulletti and colleagues[11] in 1999. The authors found a significant discrepancy in pregnancy rate for infertile women (11% with fibroids vs 25% without fibroids). Removing the fibroids increased the pregnancy rate from 25% to 42%. This study supports fibroids influence infertility.

EFFECT OF FIBROIDS ON ASSISTED REPRODUCTIVE TECHNOLOGIES

The relationship between fibroids and infertility has been elucidated through numerous studies on patients who used assisted reproductive technologies (ART), which have been summarized in several meta-analyses and systematic reviews.[12–15] Although abnormal gamete transfer and blockage of fallopian tubes are circumvented by ART, fibroids may also compromise fertility by altering the endometrial receptivity,[9,10] thus negatively affecting embryo implantation and lowering the chances for pregnancy.

Fibroid location is of critical importance in ART outcomes.[7] Submucosal fibroids, in particular, significantly reduce implantation and pregnancy rates of ART. Submucosal fibroids that distort the uterine cavity have been found to carry a relative risk of 0.3 for pregnancy and 0.28 for implantation after ART,[12,13,16] compared with infertile women without fibroids. Other authors have also demonstrated reduced success following ART with an odds ratio of 0.3 for conception and 0.3 for delivery in the presence of submucosal fibroids.[14] The effect is not as pronounced for intramural fibroids with an odds ratio of 0.62 for implantation rate and 0.7 for delivery rate per transfer cycle.[15] Similarly, Somigliana and colleagues[14] determined an odds ratio of 0.8 for conception and 0.7 for delivery with intramural fibroids. Subserosal fibroids have negligible impact on fertility with ART.[11,14]

FIBROIDS AND PREGNANCY

The reported incidence of fibroids in pregnancy ranges from 0.1% to 10.7% of all pregnancies.[17–19] A study by De Vivo and colleagues[20] reported that 71.4% of fibroids grew during the first and second trimesters, whereas 66.6% grew between the second and third trimesters. Fibroids during pregnancy are more likely to be encountered in patients who are 35 years of age and older, nulliparous, or African American.[14,18,21] Although most pregnancies with fibroids are uneventful, fibroids increase the risk of pregnancy complications.

During pregnancy, fibroids may grow quickly, causing intense pain. However, fibroid regression after live birth has been demonstrated in 72% of women, with a greater than 50% reduction in fibroid volume between early gestation and 3 to 6 months postpartum.[22] Women who had a miscarriage or used progestins after delivery experienced less fibroid regression,[22] but this difference was not present in women who delivered by cesarean, used other hormonal contraceptives, or breastfed.

A patient with fibroids who is considering pregnancy should be evaluated with a pelvic examination and an ultrasound to delineate the location and size of any fibroid(s). For patients pursuing assisted reproduction, a preconception saline infusion sonogram can be extremely helpful in such cases to identify submucosal fibroids.[4,7] Alternatively, an office hysteroscopy can be used to assess the endometrial cavity. Once a patient becomes pregnant, determining the fibroid location relative to the placenta and cervical canal may be helpful in assessing the risk of placental irregularities.

FIBROIDS AND OBSTETRIC OUTCOMES

Complications occur in approximately 10% to 40% of pregnancies in the presence of fibroids.[23,24] Fibroids may contribute to miscarriage, cesarean section, premature labor, malpresentation of the fetus, and postpartum hemorrhage (**Table 1**). Other uncommon complications include pelvic pain caused by red or carneous degeneration of the fibroid, low Apgar scores in the neonate, renal failure, fetal limb anomalies, and hypercalcemia.[25] The risk of developing complications during pregnancy increases if the fibroids are greater than 3 cm. However, women with fibroids larger than 10 cm can achieve vaginal delivery approximately 70% of the time.[18]

Table 1
Risk of obstetric outcomes in women with symptomatic uterine fibroids

Outcome	Increased Risk with Fibroids
Preterm labor	1.0–4.0
Malpresentation	1.5–4.0
Placenta previa	1.8–3.9
Placental abruption	0.5–16.5
Cesarean section	1.1–6.7
Postpartum hemorrhage	1.6–4.0
Retained placenta	2.0–2.7

All values are odds ratios unless stated otherwise.
Data from Refs.[13,24,54–56]

Fibroids clearly increase the risk of pregnancy loss. Compared with women without fibroids, women with fibroids in all locations have a relative risk of spontaneous abortion of 1.678. Women with fibroids pursuing ART also have a significantly lower ongoing pregnancy/live birth rate, with a relative risk of 0.697 compared with controls, in part because of miscarriages. Additionally, the risk of pregnancy loss correlated with fibroid location. Specifically, submucosal and intramural fibroids had notably higher rates of spontaneous abortion and notably lower rates of live births. However, subserosal fibroids had no significant impact.[12] Multiple fibroids may further increase the miscarriage rate.[13,26]

Fibroids have also been associated with malpresentation of the fetus. An odds ratio of 3.98 for breech presentation has been calculated for women with fibroids compared with women without fibroids.[17,23] Fetal malpresentation may increase the probability of a cesarean section, which subsequently increases the risk of maternal morbidity.

Last, fibroids may increase the risk of preterm labor. This is particularly true if the fibroids are large, if there are multiple fibroids, or if placentation occurs next to or overlying a fibroid. Other reports concur that fibroids increase the risk of preterm labor but do not agree on the increase in the risk of preterm birth. A 2009 meta-analysis by Olive and Pritts[12] showed no significant disparity in preterm delivery rates among patients with fibroids in all locations compared with controls.

MEDICAL THERAPIES

Current medical treatment of fibroids includes progestins, oral contraceptives, nonsteroidal anti-inflammatory drugs, tranexamic acid, and gonadotropin-releasing hormone agonists (GnRHa). Progesterone receptor agonists, selective progesterone receptor modulators, and aromatase inhibitors have also been investigated as alternatives to surgery. Some of these medical therapies are limited by undesirable side effects (**Table 2**). Progestins, nonsteroidal anti-inflammatory drugs, and oral contraceptives s have been used off-label for temporary management of bleeding; however, they are unlikely to affect fibroid volume. GnRHa reduced fibroid volume by 35% to 65% in 3 months[27] and induced amenorrhea but is typically used preoperatively to postpone surgery in a severely anemic patient or possibly to reduce uterine volume and to facilitate a vaginal approach to hysterectomy.[28] More recently, Parsanezhad and colleagues[29] reported that letrozole at 2.5 mg/d reduced fibroid size by 45.6% versus triptorelin, a GnRHa, which reduced fibroid size by only 33.2%. The antiprogestins mifepristone and ulipristal acetate also effectively induce amenorrhea and reduce fibroid volume. Donnez and colleagues[30,31] recently published 2 studies of ulipristal acetate as a treatment of fibroids. In one study, uterine bleeding was effectively controlled in 91% and 92% of women taking a 5 mg and 10 mg daily dose of ulipristal acetate, respectively, compared with 19% in women taking placebo.[31] In the second study, Donnez and colleagues[30] daily oral doses of ulipristal acetate (at both 5 mg and 10 mg) had comparable clinical outcomes and reduction in fibroid volume compared with once-monthly injections (3.75 mg) of the GnRHa leuprolide acetate. Further, this reduction was sustained for 6 months after ulipristal acetate was stopped.[30] The selective progesterone receptor modulator asoprisnil also causes a significant reduction in bleeding and size, and the effect seems to persist for 3 months.[32,33] It should be noted, however, that some of these agents have been associated with altered endometrial pathologic conditions. However, the long-term significance of the endometrial changes is not clear at present.

An effective long-term medical therapy for uterine fibroids would reduce heavy uterine bleeding and fibroid/uterine volume without excessive side effects. To date, currently approved treatments reduce symptoms only temporarily, and although new agents are in development, the ideal medical therapy has remained elusive.

MYOMECTOMY

There are different approaches to myomectomy: laparoscopically, abdominally (laparotomy), robotically, or hysteroscopically. Although myomectomies have traditionally been performed by laparotomy, the first myomectomy by laparoscopy was performed by Dr Kurt Semm in 1979. This approach eventually became mainstream in the early 1990s. Today, minimally invasive myomectomy approaches have become the preferred approach by patients and providers alike.

HYSTEROSCOPY

Submucosal fibroids, in particular, lend themselves well to a hysteroscopic surgical approach. Clinicians must determine the location, number, and percentage of the fibroids that are located in the uterine cavity. The Wamsteker classification system, used by the European Society of Gynecological Endoscopy, can be helpful in determining the probability of successful removal of submucosal fibroids by hysteroscopic myomectomy.[34] Clinicians may also use the newer STEPW (size, topography, extension, penetration, wall) classification system proposed by Lasmar and colleagues in 2005.[34] Hysteroscopic resection of submucosal fibroids offers minimal complications and rapid recovery times. Because there have been no reported cases of uterine rupture with this technique,[28] patients may attempt a vaginal delivery after hysteroscopic myomectomy.

Pregnancy Rates and Obstetric Outcomes after Myomectomy

Myomectomy is most often used for women who desire future fertility. Pregnancy rates have reached 50% to 60% after both laparoscopy and abdominal myomectomy, with good obstetric outcomes.[35] Myomectomy, however, does not eliminate symptoms permanently and is associated with surgical risks and complications (eg, loss of blood, long procedure and hospital stay, postoperative morbidity). Postoperative adhesions are of particular concern, because it is certainly possible that they may negatively impact future fertility.

Success in myomectomy depends on the location of fibroids. Intramural and subserosal fibroids are often resected using a laparoscopic or abdominal myomectomy. After undergoing an abdominal myomectomy, the risk of uterine rupture in pregnancy is low ($\sim$0.002%). Even though the incidence of uterine rupture is lower than that after a previous cesarean ($\sim$0.1%), patients with transmural incisions after abdominal or laparoscopic myomectomy generally undergo cesarean delivery.[28]

Myomectomy is of proven benefit. In a study by Casini and colleagues,[36] patients who underwent myomectomy for resection of submucosal fibroids had higher clinical pregnancy rates compared with patients with fibroids who did not undergo surgery (43.3% for operated vs 27.2% for unoperated).[36] The likelihood of live births and spontaneous abortions was similar in both groups. Summarily, data from randomized and controlled studies on the subject suggest that clinical pregnancy, live birth, and spontaneous abortion rates will normalize over time in women with submucosal fibroids after myomectomy compared with infertile women without fibroids.

Myomectomy is also beneficial for infertile patients with intramural fibroids. Casini and colleagues[36] found higher pregnancy rates in patients with intramural fibroids who underwent myomectomy, as opposed to those who did not (56.5% vs 41%,

Table 2
Summary of current medical treatment options for women with symptomatic uterine fibroids

Medications	Decreased Size/Volume	Decreased Bleeding	Side Effects	Use
Progestins	No	Yes	Induces uterine fibroid proliferation	Off-label
Oral contraceptives	No	Yes	Minimal	Off-label
Nonsteroidal anti-inflammatory drugs	No	Yes, 36% decrease found in one study[57]	Negligible	Off-label
Tranexamic acid	No	Yes		Recently approved by Food and Drug Administration, Can be used for women with or without uterine fibroids
GnRHa	Yes, 35%–65% reduction in fibroid volume, mostly occurring in the first 3 mo following treatment[27]	Yes, in 97% of patients by 6 mo. However, menses resumed in most patients 4–8 wk following discontinuation[57] Controlled uterine bleeding in 89% of patients for 3.75 mg monthly injection of leuprolide acetate[30]	Estrogen deprivation	Only preoperatively
Mifepristone	Yes, 48.1% and 39.1% reduction in fibroid volume for 5 and 10 mg dose, respectively[58]	Yes, induced amenorrhea in 60%–65% of patients[27]	Linked with endometrial thickening	Long-term use is limited by potential for endometrial hyperplasia, 28% incidence[59]

Selective progesterone receptor modulators (CDB 2914, aka ulipristal acetate)	Yes, 36% and 21% reduction in fibroid volume for 10 and 20 mg dose of CDB-2914, respectively[59] 36% and 42% median reduction in fibroid volume for 5 and 10 mg dose of ulipristal acetate, taken daily for 3 mo. This reduction was maintained for 6 mo in most patients[30]	Yes, amenorrhea in 81% and 90% of patients for 5 and 10 mg dose of CDB-2914, respectively[59] Amenorrhea in 73% and 82%, controlled bleeding in 91% and 92% of patients for 5 and 10 mg dose of ulipristal acetate, respectively, taken daily for 13 wk[31]	Linked with altered endometrial development	In Europe, ulipristal acetate is used to treat bleeding pre-operatively
Selective progesterone receptor modulators (asoprisnil)	Yes, 36% reduction in fibroid volume for 25 mg dose of asoprisnil[60]	Yes, suppressed uterine bleeding in 28%, 64%, and 83% of patients for 5, 10, and 25 mg dose of asoprisnil, respectively[60] Suppressed bleeding in 91% of patients for 25 mg dose of Asoprisnil taken for 12 wk[32]	Linked with altered endometrial morphology	
Aromatase inhibitors (eg, letrozole)	Yes, 45.6% reduction in fibroid volume[29]	No	Linked with ovarian stimulation	Off-label

Data from Refs.[27,29–32,57–60]

respectively). As stated previously, subserosal fibroids are acknowledged as having little impact on fertility.[7]

Effect of Myomectomy on ART Outcome

As discussed previously, evidence suggests that fibroid size before ART can cause lower implantation rates. In patients with intramural fibroids greater than 50 mm, myomectomy before IVF has been shown to positively impact pregnancy outcomes.[37] A study by Bulletti and colleagues[37] in 2004 compared 84 women who chose to undergo myomectomy before IVF with 84 women who started IVF but did not undergo surgery. The women who did undergo surgery had a 25% rate of delivery and a clinical pregnancy rate of 33%, compared with 12% and 15% in the nonsurgical group.[37] This study suggested that myomectomy before ART is likely to improve pregnancy outcomes in infertile patients with submucosal fibroids and with intramural fibroids greater than 5 cm.[37] For subserosal fibroids, myomectomy before ART does not affect pregnancy outcomes.

Myomectomy During Pregnancy

There is currently a lack of large, randomized, and controlled studies of the safety and efficacy of myomectomies during pregnancy and cesarean sections. Thus, myomectomy during pregnancy may be useful only in certain specific instances, such as early in pregnancy and when fibroids are large, growing rapidly, and causing recurrent pain. However, the risk of pregnancy complications including miscarriage or fetal loss is of paramount concern.

Recurrence and Reintervention after Myomectomy

Fibroid recurrence has been reported in 15% to 51% of cases up to 5 years after myomectomy.[38] This large variability was probably the result of the ethnic diversity of the study groups and of different criteria and methods used to diagnose recurrence. In the past, the probability of a subsequent surgery was thought to be based on the patient's age during the first myomectomy but may actually be more affected by parity as the cumulative probability of recurrence is decreased if a woman has children after myomectomy.

GnRHa Pretreatment Before Myomectomy

GnRHa treatment before a myomectomy has been proposed as a means to decrease fibroid volume and, thus, enhance removal while reducing complications. Vercellini and colleagues[39] showed that GnRHa pretreatment had negligible effects on blood loss, postoperative morbidity, hospital stay, and operating time. Others[27] have expressed concern that GnRHa pretreatment may increase the risk of recurrence.

MRGFUS

MRgFUS for leiomyoma treatment was approved in 2004 by the Food and Drug Administration. Initial results in symptom management are encouraging, and outcomes may be enhanced by GnRHa pretreatment.[38] Rabinovici and colleagues[40] reported 54 pregnancies in 51 women after MRgFUS, with a mean time to conception of 8 months after procedure with a 41% live birth rate. Of the women who conceived, 28% had a spontaneous abortion and 64% delivered vaginally. Of the women who delivered, there were 6.7% (1 of 15) preterm births, 2 cases of placenta previa (9%), and 93% term births.[40] Although the preliminary results are reassuring, women who become pregnant after MRgFUS should be carefully followed during pregnancy.

UAE

UAE (aka uterine fibroid embolization [UFE]) is a minimally invasive procedure that involves cutting off the blood supply of the fibroids. UFE was introduced by Ravina and colleagues[41] in 1995. In the past decade, UAE has become popular as a successful alternative to surgery. Clinical outcomes with UAE are comparable to surgery.[35] UAE offers low rates of serious complications[42–44] and rapid procedure and recovery times. Early studies have shown that 80% to 95% of patients experienced improvement in their symptoms.[42] Fibroids have also been reported to shrink by about 44% in volume in 3 months.[43] As of August 2008, the American College of Obstetricians and Gynecologists has even recognized UFE as having "level A evidence" to support that it is safe and effective in appropriately selected women.[45]

Pregnancy Rates and Obstetric Outcomes after UAE

UAE is not recommended for women with fibroids who desire future fertility, in part because of reported cases of transient and permanent amenorrhea. The reduction in menstrual flow raises the concern for endometrial damage that may contribute to abnormal placentation and/or reduced ovarian function or failure.[46] However, the incidence of amenorrhea has been found to occur in less than 5% of patients[28,44] and is clearly exacerbated by advanced age or perimenopausal status.

Goldberg and colleagues[47] suggested that pregnancies after UAE are at risk for malpresentation, preterm birth, cesarean section, and postpartum hemorrhage compared with the general population without fibroids. Homer and Sarodigan[48] found that rates of miscarriage, cesarean section, and postpartum hemorrhage were increased after UFE compared with control pregnancies with fibroids. Mara and colleagues[49] used hysteroscopy to evaluate 127 patients at 3 to 9 months after UAE (mean age 35.1 years) and found that 59.8% of the women had an abnormal endometrium with tissue necrosis (40.9%), intracavitary myoma protrusion (35.4%), endometrium "spots" (22.1%), intrauterine synechiae (10.2%), and "fistula" between the uterine cavity and intramural fibroid (6.3%). Necrosis and/or hyalinization was found in 35.4% of patients, even though 78% were asymptomatic.[49] This high rate of intrauterine pathologies after UAE may help explain the reported increased risk of in early pregnancy loss. Because UAE is still relatively new, long-term effects on fertility and pregnancy outcomes have not yet been established, and more research is needed with larger cohorts from multiple centers.

Recurrence and Reintervention after UAE

Two large randomized trials, the Randomised comparison of uterine artery embolisation (UAE) with surgical treatment in patients with symptomatic uterine fibroids (REST)[50] and Uterine artery embolization vs hysterectomy in the treatment of symptomatic uterine fibroids (EMMY)[51] trials, addressed the safety of UAE. The REST trial was composed of patients who had undergone myomectomy, hysterectomy, and UAE in the United Kingdom. Patients who had undergone surgery and UAE had similar improvements in symptoms after 5 years, but reintervention was more likely after UAE with a fibroid recurrence rate of 32%.[50] The EMMY trial, conducted in the Netherlands, compared UAE and hysterectomy, concluding that symptoms improved at similar rates for both procedures. A reintervention rate of 28% after 5 years was noted for patients who had undergone an UAE.[51]

UAE VERSUS MYOMECTOMY

Myomectomy seems to have a higher pregnancy and delivery rate than UAE or UFE. A randomized trial of 121 women conducted by Mara and colleagues[52] compared UFE to myomectomy. Two years after their procedures, 78% of the myomectomy group and 50% of the UFE group became pregnant.[52] The delivery rate was 48% and 19% and the abortion rate was 23% and 64%, for the myomectomy and UAE group, respectively.[52] Further data with longer follow-up time are needed to expound on these findings. However, Mara and colleagues[52] concluded that myomectomy seems to have better reproductive outcomes, at least in the first 2 years. Goldberg and Pereira[35] concurred that pregnancy after UFE likely yields higher rates of preterm delivery and malpresentation (odds ratio of 6.2 and 4.3, respectively) compared with laparoscopic myomectomy.

The spontaneous abortion rate found in Mara and colleagues[52] study was higher than that reported by the 2005 Ontario multicenter prospective trial (16.7%),[46] the 2005 retrospective trial of Carpenter and Walker (27%),[53] and the 2006 controlled retrospective multicenter trial of Goldberg and Pereira (24% after UAE and 15% after laparoscopic myomectomy).[35] However, all of these studies point toward the possibility that pregnant women after UAE are more likely to miscarry compared with pregnant women after myomectomy.

It should be noted that 4 women in the Mara and colleagues[52] cohort experienced reduced ovarian function. One patient had 6 weeks of amenorrhea but a normal ovarian function (follicle-stimulating hormone = 6.4 IU/L) 6 months after UAE. She subsequently became pregnant. Three women had a transient ovarian dysfunction or failure with a follicle-stimulating hormone elevation (from <10 IU/L before UAE to 15.0, 30.4, and 48.9 IU/L) accompanied by 2 months of amenorrhea in 1 patient with no response to progesterone.

UAE VERSUS MRGFUS

Rabinovici and colleagues[40] suggested that the MRgFUS term delivery rate was higher and cesarean section rate was lower than that of UAE (93% vs 71%–82%, 36% vs 50%–73%, respectively). The authors[40] also noted an increased incidence of low birth weight infants and stillbirths in women who had undergone an UAE. These obstetric complications have not been reported after MRgFUS. The time to conception, miscarriage rate, and placenta previa rate were comparable between MRgFUS and UAE.

SUMMARY

Available treatments for uterine fibroids include medical therapies, surgery, and newer options such as UAE and MRgFUS. The proper treatment of each individual patient will depend on the patient's age and desire to retain her uterus and/or future fertility. Current evidence supports that myomectomy is still the better choice for women who desire to have a child. Treatment selection will also be dictated by the location, size, and number of fibroid(s). For select women, fibroids size, previous surgery or operative risk, UFE or UAE may be the best approach.

Clinicians must balance the potential for symptom relief with associated complications of the procedure. Decisions are best founded on evidence-based efficacy of available treatment options for uterine fibroids, keeping in mind the goal of optimizing pregnancy rates and obstetric outcomes in women who desire future fertility. Designing individualized management plans will ensure optimal outcomes and maximal patient satisfaction.

ACKNOWLEDGMENTS

This research was supported, in part, by the Intramural Research Program in Reproductive and Adult Endocrinology, *Eunice Kennedy Shriver* National Institute of Child Health and Human Development, National Institutes of Health. The authors would like to thank Alan DeCherney, MD, for his mentorship and guidance and the National Institutes of Health, NICHD, PRAE, and IRTA program for their support.

REFERENCES

1. Walker C, Stewart E. Uterine fibroids: the elephant in the room. Science 2005;308: 1589–92.
2. Cramer S, Patel A. The frequency of uterine leiomyomas. Am J Clin Pathol 1990; 94:435–8.
3. Day Baird D, Dunson D, Hill M, et al. High cumulative incidence of uterine leiomyoma in black and white women: ultrasound evidence. Am J Obstet Gynecol 2003;188:100–7.
4. Ezzati M, Norian J, Segars J. Management of uterine fibroids in the patient pursuing assisted reproductive technologies. Womens Health (Lond Engl) 2009;5:413–21.
5. Peddada S, Laughlin S, Miner K, et al. Growth of uterine leiomyomata among premenopausal black and white women. Proc Natl Acad Sci U S A 2008;105: 19887–92.
6. Cardozo E, Clark A, Banks N, et al. The estimated annual cost of uterine leiomyomata in the United States. Am J Obstet Gynecol 2012;206:211.e1–9.
7. Cook H, Ezzati M, Segars J, et al. The impact of uterine leiomyomas on reproductive outcomes. Minerva Ginecol 2010;62:225–36.
8. Donnez J, Jadoul P. What are the implications of myomas on fertility? A need for a debate? Hum Reprod 2002;17:1424–30.
9. Rackow B, Taylor H. Submucosal uterine leiomyomas have a global effect on molecular determinants of endometrial receptivity. Fertil Steril 2010;93:2027–34.
10. Sinclair D, Mastroyannis A, Taylor H. Leiomyoma simultaneously impair endometrial BMP-2-mediated decidualization and anticoagulant expression through secretion of TFG-β3. J Clin Endocrinol Metab 2011;96:412–21.
11. Bulletti C, De Ziegler D, Polli V, et al. The role of leiomyomas in infertility. J Am Assoc Gynecol Laparosc 1999;6:441–5.
12. Pritts E, Parker W, Olive D. Fibroids and infertility: an updated systematic review of the evidence. Fertil Steril 2009;91:1215–23.
13. Olive D, Pritts E. Fibroids and reproduction. Semin Reprod Med 2010;28:218–27.
14. Somigliana E, Vercellini P, Daguati R, et al. Fibroids and female reproduction: a critical analysis of the evidence. Hum Reprod Update 2007;13:465–76.
15. Benecke C, Kruger T, Siebert T, et al. Effect of fibroids on fertility in patients undergoing assisted reproduction. A structured literature review. Gynecol Obstet Invest 2005;59(4):225–30.
16. Pritts E. Fibroids and infertility: a systematic review of the evidence. Obstet Gynecol Surv 2001;56:483–91.
17. Coronado G, Marshall L, Schwartz S. Complications in pregnancy, labor, and delivery with uterine leiomyomas: a population-based study. Obstet Gynecol 2000;95:764–9.
18. Qidwai G, Caughey A, Jacoby A. Obstetric outcomes in women with sonographically identified uterine leiomyomata. Obstet Gynecol 2006;107:376–82.

19. Laughlin S, Baird D, Savitz D, et al. Prevalence of uterine leiomyomas in the first trimester of pregnancy: an ultrasound-screening study. Obstet Gynecol 2009; 113:630–5.
20. De Vivo A, Mancuso A, Giacobbe A, et al. Uterine myomas during pregnancy: a longitudinal sonographic study. Ultrasound Obstet Gynecol 2011;37:361–5.
21. Stout M, Odibo A, Graseck A, et al. Leiomyomas at routine second trimester ultrasound examination and adverse obstetric outcomes. Obstet Gynecol 2010;116: 1056–63.
22. Laughlin S, Hartmann K, Baird D. Postpartum factors and natural fibroid regression. Am J Obstet Gynecol 2011;204:496.
23. Ouyang DW, Economy KE, Norwitz ER. Obstetric complications of fibroids. Obstet Gynecol Clin North Am 2006;33:153–69.
24. Exacoustòs C, Rosati P. Ultrasound diagnosis of uterine myomas and complications in pregnancy. Obstet Gynecol 1993;82:97–101.
25. Johnson NL, Norwitz E, Segars JH. Management of fibroids in pregnancy. In: Fibroids: gynecology in practice. Oxford (United Kingdom): Wiley-Blackwell; in press.
26. Lee H, Norwitz E, Shaw J. Contemporary management of fibroids in pregnancy. Rev Obstet Gynecol 2010;3:20–38.
27. Olive D, Lindheim S, Pritts E. Non-surgical management of leiomyoma: impact on fertility. Curr Opin Obstet Gynecol 2004;16:239–43.
28. Stewart E. Uterine fibroids. Lancet 2001;357:293–8.
29. Parsanezhad M, Azmoon M, Alborzi S, et al. A randomized, controlled clinical trial comparing the effects of aromatase inhibitor (letrozole) and gonadotropin-releasing hormone agonist (triptorelin) on uterine leiomyoma volume and hormonal status. Fertil Steril 2010;93:192–8.
30. Donnez J, Tomaszewski J, Vazquez F, et al. Ulipristal acetate versus leuprolide acetate for uterine fibroids. N Engl J Med 2012;366:421–32.
31. Donnez J, Tatarchuk T, Bouchard P, et al. Ulipristal acetate versus placebo for fibroid treatment before surgery. N Engl J Med 2012;366:409–20.
32. Wilkens J, Chwalisz K, Han C, et al. Effects of the selective progesterone receptor modulator asoprisnil on uterine artery blood flow, ovarian activity, and clinical symptoms in patients with uterine leiomyomata scheduled for hysterectomy. J Clin Endocrinol Metab 2008;93:4664–71.
33. Williams A, Critchley H, Osei J, et al. The effects of the selective progesterone receptor modulator asoprisnil on the morphology of uterine tissues after 3 month treatment in patients with symptomatic uterine leiomyomata. Hum Reprod 2007; 22:1696–704.
34. Lasmar R, Xinmei Z, Indman P, et al. Feasibility of a new classification of submucous myomas: a multicenter study. Fertil Steril 2011;95:2773–7.
35. Goldberg J, Pereira L. Pregnancy outcomes following treatment for fibroids: uterine fibroid embolization versus laparoscopic myomectomy. Curr Opin Obstet Gynecol 2006;18:402–6.
36. Casini M, Rossi F, Agostini R, et al. Effects of the position of fibroids on fertility. Gynecol Endocrinol 2006;22:106–9.
37. Bulletti C, DE Ziegler D, Levi Setti P, et al. Myomas, pregnancy outcome, and in vitro fertilization. Ann N Y Acad Sci 2004;1034:84–92.
38. Al Hilli M, Stewart E. Magnetic resonance-guided focused ultrasound surgery. Semin Reprod Med 2010;28:242–9.
39. Vercellini P, Trespidi L, Zaina B, et al. Gonadotropin-releasing hormone agonist treatment before abdominal myomectomy: a controlled trial. Fertil Steril 2003; 79:1390–5.

40. Rabinovici J, David M, Fukunishi H, et al. Pregnancy outcome after magnetic resonance-guided focused ultrasound surgery (MRgFUS) for conservative treatment of uterine fibroids. Fertil Steril 2010;93(1):199–209.
41. Ravina J, Herbreteau C, Ciracu-Vigneron N, et al. Arterial embolization to treat uterine myomata. Lancet 1995;346:671–2.
42. Freed M, Spies J. Uterine artery embolization for fibroids: a review of current outcomes. Semin Reprod Med 2010;28:235–41.
43. Spies J, Ascher S, Roth A, et al. Uterine artery embolization for leiomyomata. Obstet Gynecol 2001;98:29–34.
44. Spies J, Roth A, Gonsalves S, et al. Ovarian function after uterine artery embolization for leiomyomata: assessment with use of serum follicle stimulating hormone assay. J Vasc Interv Radiol 2001;12:437–42.
45. American College of Obstetricians and Gynecologists. ACOG practice bulletin: alternatives to hysterectomy in the management of leiomyomas. Obstet Gynecol 2008;112:387–400.
46. Pron G, Mocarski E, Bennett J, et al. Pregnancy after uterine artery embolization for leiomyomata: the Ontario multicenter trial. Obstet Gynecol 2005;105:67–76.
47. Goldberg J, Pereira L, Berghella V. Pregnancy after uterine artery embolization. Obstet Gynecol 2002;100(5):869–72.
48. Homer H, Sarodigan E. Uterine artery embolization for fibroids is associated with an increased risk of miscarriage. Fertil Steril 2010;92:324–30.
49. Mara M, Horak P, Kubinova K, et al. Hysteroscopy after uterine fibroid embolization: evaluation of intrauterine findings in 127 patients. J Obstet Gynaecol Res 2012;38(5):823–31.
50. Moss J, Cooper K, Khaund A, et al. Randomised comparison of uterine artery embolisation (UAE) with surgical treatment in patients with symptomatic uterine fibroids (REST trial): 5-year results. BJOG 2011;118:936–44.
51. van der Kooij S, Hehenkamp W, Volkers N, et al. Uterine artery embolization vs hysterectomy in the treatment of symptomatic uterine fibroids: 5-year outcome from the randomized EMMY trial. Am J Obstet Gynecol 2010;203:105.e1–105.e13.
52. Mara M, Maskova J, Fucikova Z, et al. Midterm clinical and first reproductive results of a randomized controlled trial comparing uterine fibroid embolization and myomectomy. Cardiovasc Intervent Radiol 2008;31:73–85.
53. Carpenter T, Walker W. Pregnancy following uterine artery embolization for symptomatic fibroids: a series of 26 completed pregnancies. BJOG 2005;11:321–5.
54. Klatsky P, Tran N, Caughey A, et al. Fibroids and reproductive outcomes: a systematic literature review from conception to delivery. Am J Obstet Gynecol 2008;198:357–66.
55. Vergani P, Locatelli A, Ghidini A, et al. Large uterine leiomyomas and risk of cesarean delivery. Obstet Gynecol 2007;109:410–4.
56. Rice J, Kay H, Mahony B. The clinical significance of uterine leiomyomas in pregnancy. Am J Obstet Gynecol 1989;160:1212–6.
57. Parker W. Uterine myomas: management. Fertil Steril 2007;88:255–71.
58. Esteve J, Acosta R, Pérez Y, et al. Treatment of uterine myoma with 5 or 10 mg mifepristone during 6 months, post-treatment evolution over 12 months: double-blind randomized clinical trial. Eur J Obstet Gynecol Reprod Biol 2012;161:202–8.
59. Levens E, Potlog-Nahari C, Armstrong A, et al. CDB-2914 for uterine leiomyomata treatment: a randomized controlled trial. Obstet Gynecol 2008;111:1129–36.
60. Chwalisz K, Larsen L, Mattia-Goldberg C, et al. A randomized, controlled trial of asoprisnil, a novel selective progesterone receptor modulator, in women with uterine leiomyomata. Fertil Steril 2007;87:1399–412.

Endometriosis and Infertility

A Review of the Pathogenesis and Treatment of Endometriosis-associated Infertility

Matthew Latham Macer, MD, Hugh S. Taylor, MD*

KEYWORDS

- Endometriosis • Infertility • Treatment • Pathogenesis • Stem cell
- In vitro fertilization

KEY POINTS

- Endometriosis is an estrogen-dependent disease that affects between 10% and 15% of reproductive-age women.
- There is a well-established association between endometriosis and infertility; however, causes seem to be multifactorial, involving mechanical, molecular, genetics, and environmental causes.
- The optimal method for treatment of endometriosis-associated infertility is an individualized decision that should be made on patient-specific basis.
- In vitro fertilization is currently the most effective treatment of endometriosis-associated infertility.

Endometriosis has been estimated to affect up to 10% to 15% of reproductive-age women.[1] The association between endometriosis and infertility is well supported throughout the literature, but a definite cause-effect relationship is still controversial. The prevalence of endometriosis increases dramatically to as high as 25% to 50% in women with infertility, and 30% to 50% of women with endometriosis have infertility.[2] The fecundity rate in normal reproductive-age couples without infertility is estimated to be around 15% to 20%, whereas the fecundity rate in women with untreated endometriosis is estimated to range from 2% to 10%.[3,4] Women with mild endometriosis have been shown to have a significantly lower probability of pregnancy during a period of 3 years than do women with unexplained fertility (36% vs 55%, respectively).[5] In vitro fertilization (IVF) studies have suggested that women with more advanced endometriosis have poor ovarian reserve, low oocyte and embryo quality, and poor implantation.[6,7]

Department of Obstetrics, Gynecology and Reproductive Sciences, Yale School of Medicine, 333 Cedar Street, PO Box 208063, New Haven, CT 06520-8063, USA
* Corresponding author.
E-mail address: hugh.taylor@yale.edu

Obstet Gynecol Clin N Am 39 (2012) 535–549
http://dx.doi.org/10.1016/j.ogc.2012.10.002
0889-8545/12/$ – see front matter © 2012 Elsevier Inc. All rights reserved.

Despite the well-supported association between endometriosis and infertility, the difficulty in proving a causal relationship likely stems from the multiple mechanisms by which endometriosis can impact fertility and the heterogeneity and variations in the phenotype of the disease. This article will discuss endometriosis-associated infertility including a basic background on endometriosis, its presumed pathophysiology in causing infertility, and both current and potential treatments.

ENDOMETRIOSIS: OVERVIEW

Endometriosis is an estrogen-dependent benign inflammatory disease characterized by the presence of ectopic endometrial implants.[8] Implants typically occur in the pelvis but have also been seen in the upper abdomen, peripheral and axial skeleton, lungs, diaphragm, and central nervous system. The most common sites of endometriosis, in decreasing order, are the ovaries, anterior/posterior cul-de-sac, broad ligaments and uterosacral ligaments, uterus, fallopian tubes, sigmoid colon, and appendix.

Because the growth of the implants depends on ovary-produced steroids, it is a disease that most severely affects women ages 25 to 35 years.[9] Patients can present with a wide range of symptoms, from being asymptomatic to infertile. In addition to infertility, it is commonly associated with symptoms such as dyspareunia, dysmenorrhea, bladder/bowel symptoms, and chronic pelvic pain.

PATHOGENESIS OF ENDOMETRIOSIS

The definite pathogenesis of endometriosis is still unknown but there are several leading theories, including retrograde menstruation, altered immunity, coelomic metaplasia, and metastatic spread. Newer research is also proposing stem cell and genetic origins of the disease.

Retrograde Menstruation

The most well-accepted theory, retrograde menstruation, was proposed by Sampson in the 1920s and states that endometrial tissue is transported in a retrograde fashion through patent fallopian tubes into the peritoneal cavity.[8,10] The endometrial cells then attach to the peritoneal mesothelial cells, establish a blood supply, proliferate, and produce endometrial implants. This theory has been well supported by subsequent research. Women with endometriosis have higher volumes of refluxed menstrual blood and endometrial-tissue fragments than do women without the disorder.[11] In addition, endometriosis is observed when the cervix of baboons is ligated and endometrial fragments have access to the pelvis.[12] The incidence of endometriosis is much higher in young girls with outflow obstruction, thereby leading to increased tubal reflux and retrograde menstruation.[13] However, the incidence of retrograde menstruation is similar in women with and without endometriosis, so the pathogenesis seems to be a multifactorial mechanism.

Coelomic Metaplasia and Metastatic Spread

In the 1960s, Ferguson and colleagues proposed that coelomic metaplasia may also contribute to the development of endometriosis. It stems from the theory that the peritoneum contains undifferentiated cells that can differentiate into endometrial cells.[14] Another theory argues that menstrual tissue travels from the endometrial cavity through lymphatic channels and veins to distant sites, which could attribute to implants found outside the pelvic cavity.

Altered Immunity

Women with endometriosis have altered immunity, preventing them from clearing the refluxed endometrial cells/fragments that appear in retrograde menstruation.[15] This would help explain why some women with retrograde menstruation develop endometriosis, whereas others do not. Cell-mediated immunity is thought to be deficient in patients with the disease; leukocytes are unable to recognize that the endometrial tissue is not in its normal location.[15] There have also been studies showing decreased cytotoxicity to endometrial cells secondary to defective natural killer cell activity.[16] Once endometriosis develops, the immune system has also been to shown to potentiate the development and increase the severity of the disease. In women with endometriosis, there are increased numbers of leukocytes and macrophages in and around endometrial implants and in the peritoneal fluid. These cells secrete cytokines and growth factors (interleukins 1, 6, and 8; tumor necrosis factor; RANTES, vascular endothelial growth factor [VEGF]) into the peritoneal milieu, which then recruit surrounding capillaries and leukocytes.[17–19] The ultimate effect is proliferation of endometriosis implants with increased vascular supply.

In addition to retrograde menstruation, coelomic metaplasia, and altered immunity, newer research is increasingly showing that stem cells and genetics may play a role in causing endometriosis.

Stem Cells

It is presumed that de novo development of endometrial tissue occurs from endogenous stem cells in the endometrium.[20,21] During the past decade, we have studied the possibility that bone marrow–derived cells may also differentiate into endometrial cells and, pertinently, may be implicated in the development of ectopic endometrial implants. If true, this would help explain how ectopic tissue can occur in locations outside the peritoneal cavity such as the lung and central nervous systems. Proof that endometrial cells can be derived from bone marrow mesenchymal stem cells comes from the study of female allogenic bone marrow transplant recipients who received marrow from a single antigen-mismatched related donor, allowing the cells to be identifiable by human leukocyte antigen type. The study remarkably showed the presence of donor-derived endometrial cells in endometrial biopsies of the recipients.[22] This finding suggested that bone marrow–derived stem cells can differentiate into human uterine endometrium. An additional study in 2007 used a murine model and transplanted male donor–derived bone marrow cells into female bone marrow.[21] After transplantation, male donor–derived bone marrow cells (recognizable by the Y chromosome) were found in the uterine endometrium and had differentiated into both epidermal and stromal cells. This is evidence that bone-marrow stem cells from male donors can generate endometrium de novo and proves their mesenchymal origin. This study also showed the ability of stem cells to engraft endometriosis by showing the presence of bone marrow–derived cells in ectopic endometrial implants in previously hysterectomized mice. The endometrial tissue must be capable of attracting stem cells despite its ectopic location. This evidence shows that a nonendometrial stem cell source can result in endometrial cells in both the uterus and ectopic implants. This suggests an alternative origin of some endometriosis, specifically, from bone marrow–derived cells.[21]

Genetics

For more than 20 years, it has been known that endometriosis has a familial tendency. Women who have a first-degree relative affected by the disease have a 7-times higher risk of developing endometriosis than women who do not have a family history of the disease.[23] Familial aggregation has also been shown in studies of monozygotic twins and studies involving nonhuman primates.[24,25] Genetic polymorphisms may lead to aberrantly expressed genes identified in the endometrium of both human and nonhuman primates, but their contribution to the cause of endometriosis is not yet well defined.[26-28] Alternatively, these alterations in gene expression are more likely acquired and indeed are seen in animal models of the disease in which normal endometrium (without genetic predisposition to the disease) is transplanted to the peritoneal cavity.[29,30]

The only mouse model of spontaneous endometriosis is obtained by engineering the expression of an oncogenic variant of the KRAS gene.[31] KRAS is a signal transduction molecule that is mutated in several cancers and can lead to increased cell proliferation, survival, and migration. Mice expressing this gene develop spontaneous endometriosis. Recently, a polymorphism in the KRAS gene has been reported in a group of women with resistant endometriosis.[32] Specific genetic alterations may allow the identification of endometriosis subtypes, which may allow risk stratification, individualized therapy, and personalized medicine for endometriosis.

ENDOMETRIOSIS-ASSOCIATED INFERTILITY

Here we discuss the current evidence and proposed mechanisms regarding how endometriosis adversely impacts fertility. It is clear how severe disease can cause infertility. Pelvic anatomy becomes distorted and fecundity is reduced via mechanical disruptions such as pelvic adhesions. These disruptions impair oocyte release or pickup, alter sperm motility, cause disordered myometrial contractions, and impair fertilization and embryo transport.[33] Women who are infertile are more likely to have advanced stages of the disease.[34] However, there is still much speculation about the proposed mechanisms by which mild disease impacts fertility.[1] Inflammatory cytokines, growth and angiogenic factors, and aberrantly expressed genes are all being explored as potential etiologic factors of endometriosis-associated infertility.

Effect on Gametes and Embryo

Altered ovulation and oocyte production are seen in endometriosis and are associated with the increased inflammatory cells in the peritoneal fluid and endometriomas. Inflammatory effects resulting from the presence of endometriomas have been shown to affect both oocyte production and ovulation in the affected ovary.[33] There is also a luteal phase disruption in endometriosis that may result from progesterone receptor dysregulation and an effect on progesterone target genes, which in turn leads to decreased endometrial receptivity.[8,33] Sperm quality or function is also decreased and has been proposed to result from the inflammatory/toxic affects of the peritoneal fluid and increased activated macrophages.[35] The increased number of inflammatory cells in the peritoneal fluid not only damage the oocytes and sperm but have also been shown to have toxic effects on the embryo.[36] In addition, studies have shown aberrant expression of glutathione peroxidase and catalase in the endometrium of patients with endometriosis and it can be suspected that there is also an increase in endometrial free radicals and subsequently a negative effect on embryo viability.[37,38]

Effect on Fallopian Tube and Embryo Transport

Gamete transport is also affected by the inflammatory environment and increased cytokines found in endometriosis; inflammation impairs tubal function and decreases tubal motility. Disordered myometrial contractions associated with endometriosis can also impair gamete transport and embryo implantation.[33]

Effect on the Endometrium

In addition to the mentioned inflammatory effects of endometriosis, there is increasing evidence supporting that endometriosis affects the eutopic endometrium and causes implantation failure; however, the mechanism of cellular or molecular signaling from the lesion to the uterus is unknown. As described, numerous genes are aberrantly expressed in the endometrium of women with endometriosis, many known to be necessary for endometrial receptivity. The mechanism and specific signal that lead to alterations in the endometrium of women with endometriosis are not well characterized. We recently published data demonstrating that cells migrate from ectopic endometrial implants to the eutopic endometrium.[39] Experimental endometriosis was established by implanting endometrial tissue from green fluorescent protein (GFP) mice into the peritoneal cavity of DS-Red mice. The study showed that GFP-positive cells were found in the eutopic endometrium, preferentially the basalis layer, of mice with experimental endometriosis. In addition, gene expression profiling of the GFP-positive cells showed increased expression of pan-epithelial markers and, more interestingly, upregulation of *Wnt7A* expression along with 17 other genes in the *wingless pathway*. *Wnt7a* is essential to estrogen-mediated uterine growth and implantation in mice, likely by signaling between the epithelium and stroma.[40–42] It has been theorized by Liu and colleagues[43] that aberrant activation of the *Wnt* pathway disturbs endometrial development during the implantation window. We theorize that the increased expression of ectopic *Wnt7a* outside of the gland likely disrupts the normal epithelial-stromal polarity required for normal fertility.[39] There is likely bidirectional movement of cells between the eutopic and ectopic endometrial tissue. The reprogrammed and abnormally located cells likely that have "returned" to the endometrium generate the signal that leads to aberrant gene expression and implantation failure.

There are several other studies proposing that aberrant gene expression in eutopic and ectopic endometrium may be related to infertility or the establishment of the disease.

An example of aberrant gene expression is the *Hoxa10/HOXA10* gene.[27] This gene is directly involved in the embryogenesis of the uterus and subsequently in endometrial regeneration in each menstrual cycle. Expression of this gene is necessary for endometrial receptivity. Mice with a targeted disruption of the *Hoxa10* gene show complete loss of endometrial receptivity. Similarly, women with lower levels of expression of *HOXA10* have lower implantation rates. In women, cyclical endometrial expression of this gene peaks during the window of implantation in response to estrogen and progesterone. Women with endometriosis, however, do not exhibit the mid-luteal rise as would be expected, which may partially explain their infertility.[28]

Aromatase, the enzyme that converts androstenedione and testosterone to estrone and estradiol, has also been extensively studied in endometriosis. It has been shown that abnormal levels of aromatase are present in both endometriotic implants and eutopic endometrium, where it is normally absent, resulting in increased estradiol production.[44] The role of aromatase in the pathophysiology of endometriosis is clear given that it is an estrogen-dependent disease; increased estrogen production in the endometrium may also affect endometrial development and receptivity.

Progesterone resistance and dysregulation of progesterone receptors also seem to play a role in implantation failure. Because progesterone induces endometrial decidualization during the luteal phase, its presence is crucial for a normal pregnancy. Progesterone receptors have been shown to be dysregulated in both eutopic and ectopic endometrium. Down-regulation of receptors is seen before implantation in normal endometrium but is delayed in the endometrium of endometriosis.[45] In addition, both eutopic and ectopic endometrium have been shown to be resistant to progesterone, causing an unopposed estrogen state that is likely not suitable for implantation.[46,47]

Recent studies have also shown an association with the abnormal progesterone resistance and inappropriately persistent expression of matrix metalloproteinases, which degrade extracellular matrices.[48] Matrix metalloproteinases are normally inhibited by progesterone in the secretory phase, but in the setting of endometriosis, they remain elevated during inappropriate periods such as implantation. The disinhibition of these proteins could theoretically lead to an environment of constant matrix breakdown not conducive to implantation.

Around the same time that progesterone receptors are downregulated during implantation, epithelial expression of αβ-integrin, a marker of uterine receptivity, is normally increased.[49] Patients with endometriosis have lower expression of this adhesion molecule, which may interfere with embryo attachment in implantation.[8,49]

There is a well-established association between endometriosis and infertility; however, as shown here earlier, it seems to be multifactorial, involving mechanical, molecular, genetics, and environmental causes. As newer research identifies alterations in gene expression and genetic defects, it is appropriate to consider testing of endometrial adequacy to diagnose and treat endometriosis-associated infertility.

TREATMENT OF ENDOMETRIOSIS-ASSOCIATED INFERTILITY

Current treatment of endometriosis-associated infertility focuses on improving fecundity by removing or reducing ectopic endometrial implants and restoring normal pelvic anatomy.[50] A wide spectrum of treatment options have been examined, including expectant management, medical treatment, surgical treatment, and assisted reproductive technology (ART). Current research is also examining novel promising nonhormonal treatment options for endometriosis such as immunoconjugate, VEGF antagonists, and stem cells, which may also prove to increase fecundity by decreasing the extent of ectopic implants or improving the eutopic endometrium.[51,52]

Expectant Management

Despite the significantly lower fecundity rate compared with women without endometriosis, women with mild-moderate endometriosis are still able to conceive in the absence of any medical or surgical intervention. Multiple studies evaluating patients with endometriosis who undergo expectant management report their fecundity rate to be around 2.40 to 3.0 per 100 person-months.[53,54] However, in women with more severe disease, pregnancy rates are far lower.[50] Although the option of expectant management may be reasonable for patients with mild-moderate disease, it is only delaying the start of effective treatment in those with severe disease. Patient counseling must take into account the severity of endometriosis.

Medical Treatment

It is well known that endometriosis is an estrogen-dependent disorder. Endometriotic lesions have been shown to have an increased production and decreased inactivation of estradiol. This is due, in part, to abnormal expression of both aromatase and 17β-hydroxysteroid dehydrogenase.[44,55] Common medical therapies used to treat symptoms of endometriosis such as pelvic pain, dyspareunia, and dysmenorrhea target ovarian estrogen production. Medications used as endometriosis therapy are hormonal medications and include combined oral contraceptives, progestins, danazol and gonadotropin-releasing hormone agonists or antagonists (GnRH analogs). Although these medications may help treat pain, they have shown no benefit in the treatment of endometriosis-associated infertility. A 2010 Cochrane review looked at 25 trials of ovulation-suppressive agents (danazol, progestins, oral contraceptives, GnRH agonists) in women with endometriosis-associated infertility who wished to conceive. The odds ratios (ORs) for pregnancy following ovulation suppression versus placebo or no treatment was 0.97 (95% confidence interval [CI] 0.68–1.34, $P = .8$) for all women randomized and 1.02 (95% CI 0.70–1.52, $P = .82$) for subfertile couples.[56] Not only was there no benefit from ovulation suppression, but it also delayed the patient from having a live birth while taking the suppressive agents.

We recently reviewed several novel medical therapies being tested for the treatment of endometriosis.[51] Some are hormonal, such as selective estrogen receptor modulators and selective progesterone receptor modulators, whereas others target inflammation and angiogenesis such as statins, VEGF receptor antagonists, and immunoconjugate. Other trends in the treatment of endometriosis include the use of aromatase inhibitors, cyclooxygenase-2 inhibitors, omega-3 fatty acids, and cannabinoid agonists.[57] Despite increasing research on the novel therapies, evidence to date is primarily limited to experimental animal models; further trials in women will be needed to define their role and utility in endometriosis-associated infertility.

As a general rule, medical therapy should be discouraged in patients with endometriosis and subfertility who desire a live birth.[50] The exception to this rule is in patients undergoing in vitro fertilization (IVF). Multiple studies have shown that prolonged GnRH agonist treatment before IVF may improve fertility rates in advanced endometriosis.[58–60] Proposed mechanisms are via increased retrieved oocytes, higher implantation rates, and reduced preclinical abortions.[61,62] A Cochrane review looked at 3 randomized controlled trials and concluded that the administration of GnRH agonists for a period of 3 to 6 months before IVF or intracytoplasmic sperm injection (ICSI) in women with endometriosis significantly increases the odds of a clinical pregnancy (OR 4.28, 95% CI 2.00–9.15).[63] Similar to GnRH agonists, the use of oral contraceptives has been shown to improve outcomes when given for 6 to 8 weeks before ART. A randomized controlled trial by de Ziegler and colleagues[64] showed outcomes comparable to age-matched controls of women who did not have endometriosis.

Data regarding GnRH and OCP therapy in patients with endometriomas has however remained controversial. A 2010 Cochran review by Benschop and colleagues[65] concluded that administration of GnRHa does not significantly affect the clinical pregnancy rate when given before ART in patients with endometriomas; however, there was improved ovarian response and a greater number of mature oocytes were aspirated. Conversely, the study by de Ziegler and colleagues[64] showed improvement using pre-ART continuous oral contraceptive therapy for 6 to 8 weeks even in those with endometriomas. Data regarding suppressive therapy before ART in patients with endometriomas are still evolving but show promise for improving endometriosis-related infertility when used in conjunction with IVF.

In women with moderate-severe endometriosis, prolonged GnRH agonist administration should be considered before IVF.[66] It is also reasonable to consider the use of continuous oral contraceptive therapy before ART in patients with all stages of endometriosis.

Surgical Treatment

Surgery for endometriosis can be both diagnostic and therapeutic. Laparoscopic surgery is preferred to laparotomy; it is more cost effective and has a shorter hospital stay and shorter recovery.[67] Surgical treatment of endometriosis-associated infertility has proposed benefits in both severe and minimal-moderate disease. Benefits of surgery in severe disease include restoration of pelvic anatomy, removal of implants and endometriomas, and resulting decreased inflammation. There are few randomized controlled trials studying the effects of surgery on fecundity in advanced-stage disease, and there is insufficient evidence to recommend surgery for the treatment of infertility in severe disease. However, as long as ovarian resection is limited to avoid substantial reduction in ovarian reserve, surgery in severe disease should remain an option in patients with severe endometriosis-associated infertility who desire a live birth. Surgery in minimal-moderate disease is a little more controversial, but evidence to date supports surgical intervention. Marcoux and colleagues[53] conducted a randomized controlled trial with 341 women to determine whether laparoscopic surgery enhanced fecundity in infertile women with minimal-mild endometriosis. They concluded that either resection or ablation of minimal and mild endometriosis significantly enhanced fecundity in infertile women compared with diagnostic laparoscopy alone (cumulative probabilities, 30.7% and 17.7%, respectively; $P = .006$). The corresponding fecundity rates were 4.7 and 2.4 per 100 person-months, respectively, and the absolute increase in the 36-week probability of a pregnancy carried beyond 20 weeks that was attributable to surgery was 13%. They also showed no significant difference between excisional versus ablative techniques. However, contradictory evidence was seen in an Italian study of similar design but with a smaller number of subjects that found no significant difference in conception rates.[68] A subsequent meta-analysis that was later reaffirmed by a Cochrane review concluded that surgery had significant benefits in infertile patients with early-stage endometriosis who desired fertility. The number of women who needed to undergo laparoscopic surgery for one additional clinical pregnancy was approximately 7.7 and the OR was 1.66 (95% CI 1.09–2.51) in favor of laparoscopic surgery versus diagnostic surgery only.[69,70] However, given the relatively small increase in pregnancy, alternative therapies should also be considered.

Studies on the treatment of an endometrioma in the setting of infertility are more uniform. A 2008 Cochrane review examined the current literature regarding laparoscopic ablation versus excision of endometriomas and found that excision of the cyst was associated with a subsequent increased spontaneous pregnancy rate in women who had documented prior subfertility (OR 5.21, 95% CI 2.04–13.29). Resection was clearly superior compared with drainage or ablation. This review also identified a randomized controlled trial that demonstrated an increased ovarian follicular response to gonadotropin in those who underwent excisional surgery compared with ablative surgery.[71] In addition, excisional surgery was associated with a reduced rate of recurrence and superior improvement in pain.

Combined Medical and Surgical Treatment

Many studies have looked at combined medical and surgical therapies, specifically, preoperative and postoperative medical therapy. Preoperative medical therapy was administered with the intent of reducing the severity of endometriosis and thereby decreasing the risk and increasing the desired outcome of the surgery. Although the preoperative use of a GnRH agonist can reduce the severity of disease, there is no convincing evidence that it impacts surgical success or fertility rate.[50,72,73] Likewise, multiple randomized trials have evaluated the use of ovarian suppression postoperatively. The aim was to increase resorption of residual deposits and reduce the recurrence of disease; however, no trial reported increased fertility rates.[59] A 2009 Cochrane review looked at 16 trials of preoperative or postoperative hormonal suppression and found that there was no evidence of benefit associated with postsurgical medical therapy and insufficient evidence to determine a benefit to preoperative therapy with regard to pain, disease recurrence, or pregnancy rates.[74] Given these studies, adjuvant medical therapy is not recommended.

Superovulation and Intrauterine Insemination

Multiple randomized controlled trials have shown that ovulation induction and superovulation both with and without intrauterine insemination (IUI) increase fertility rates in patients without distorted anatomy.[75–78] All of these studies focused on patients with minimal-mild endometriosis. There is a lack of data for patients with more advanced endometriosis. Guznick showed that fecundity rates were highest when combining gonadotropin induction with IUI compared with the use of intracervical insemination (ICI) or IUI/ICI alone.[76] Another study suggested benefit with clomiphene citrate and IUI compared with controls (fecundity 0.095 vs 0.033).[79] In addition, a recent randomized study comparing IUI with clomiphene versus IUI with letrozole showed a benefit in clinical pregnancy rates with either (14.7 vs 15.9%, respectively) in women with surgically treated minimal-mild endometriosis and no difference between the 2 methods.[80] An important aspect to remember is that ovarian stimulation can also exacerbate endometriosis, so it should be performed in a controlled manner and be limited to 3 or 4 cycles.[50,81] To summarize, there is evidence to support superovulation/IUI in women with stage I or II endometriosis, especially if they have been surgically diagnosed and shown to be free of anatomic distortion before the therapy. There is insufficient evidence to support superovulation/IUI in patients with severe endometriosis.

ART

IVF is currently the most effective treatment of endometriosis-associated infertility. The Society of Assisted Reproductive Technology reported that in 2009, more than 1400 live births were reported from 5600 IVF cycles in patients with endometriosis. However, when comparing data on the effectiveness of IVF for patients with endometriosis versus patients with other causes of infertility, there is still controversy. A recent report on the Society of Assisted Reproductive Technology data showed that the average delivery rate per retrieval of patient's undergoing IVF–embryo transfer was 39.1% for women with endometriosis compared with 33.2% for women with all causes of infertility. This suggests that women with endometriosis seem to have similar or even slightly increased success in IVF compared with women with other causes of infertility.[82] Additionally, a study by Opoien and colleagues[83] showed that excluding women with endometriomas, women with all stages of endometriosis who underwent luteal phase GnRH agonist down-regulation followed by IVF/ICSI treatment had a similar pregnancy and live birth rate compared with women with tubal factor infertility. Patients with endometriomas, however, did show a significantly lower pregnancy and live birth rate. Similarly, an analysis of the Human Fertilization and Embryology database suggested that live birth rates were not affected by endometriosis compared with unexplained infertility.[50] Additionally, a study by Bukulmez and colleagues showed that no evidence suggests that the presence or extent of endometriosis affects the clinical pregnancy or implantation rate in patients that are undergoing ICSI.[84]

To summarize, although it is still uncertain how much endometriosis affects IVF success rates, IVF seems to be the most successful treatment option for patients with all stages of endometriosis. In addition, it is not unreasonable to consider pretreatment ovulation suppression to help suppress inflammatory cytokines and reduce disease presence before any form of ART. In patients with endometriomas, more research is needed to assess their affect on IVF/ICSI and whether surgical intervention before ART increases their success rate.

Potential Treatments in the Future

There are several novel medical therapies, as mentioned earlier, that are currently being examined for use in endometriosis and a few show potential as a medical therapy in endometriosis-associated infertility. These include but are not limited to immunoconjugate and aromatase inhibitors. Immunoconjugate targets aberrantly expressed tissue factor on endometriotic endothelium and prompts regression of the established disease, likely via devascularization.[51] It has the potential to destroy preexisting implants in a nontoxic, nonhormonal manner, which could subsequently improve fertility rates. Aromatase inhibitors are another potential treatment. As described, aromatase is found in eutopic endometrium, where it is normally absent, and may impact estradiol levels and implantation. Aromatase inhibitors are being increasingly studied for the use of endometriosis-associated pain, but clinical trials studying their potential with current fertility treatments are still needed.

As discussed, there is currently ongoing research on the impact both genetics and stem cells may have on endometriosis. The HOXA10 gene has been implicated in the pathogenesis of endometriosis-associated infertility by affecting implantation.[27] There is evidence that epigenetic modifications may play a larger role than once believed. Epigenetics is the alteration of DNA by long-lasting covalent modification such as the addition of a methyl group but without a mutation or change in any base pair. These epigenetic changes have been described in numerous studies including hypermethylation of HOXA10, progesterone receptor-β, and E-cadherin or hypomethylation of genes for estrogen receptor-β and steroidogenic factor 1.[77,85] Potential future treatments could involve targeting these altered molecular pathways and correcting abnormal methylation. Unfortunately, there are no safe and effective ways currently available to correct these defects. Replacement of endometrium is a potential option. Stem cell therapies (discussed later) are a potential option to replace damaged endometrium.

Finally, some of the newest data show great potential as future treatment strategies. We have previously shown that bone marrow–derived mesenchymal stem cells can give rise to endometrial cells; in addition, there is likely a bidirectional communication between eutopic endometrium and endometrial implants. This information could help to foster a better understanding of the disease, and knowledge of this process could lead to potential therapies for treating uterine disorders and therapeutically augmenting stem cell transdifferentiation into endometrium. Damaged endometrium can be replaced with stem cells. This is especially appealing given the epigenetic damage to endometrium seen in women with endometriosis; epigenetic alterations are persistent and there are no known therapies to reverse this damage. Replacement of endometrium with a stem cell–based therapy may be the optimal way to restore normal endometrial function and implantation in women with endometriosis.

Summary of Treatment Options

Ultimately, the optimal method for treatment of endometriosis-associated infertility is an individualized decision that should be made on patient-specific basis. Many factors must be taken into account including but not limited to distorted pelvic anatomy, patient's ovarian reserve, partner semen analysis, age, presence of endometriomas, and length of infertility.[77] Depending on the patient, current treatment options may include expectant management, surgical removal of implants, ovulation induction or IVF. For women with suspected stage I/II endometriosis, a decision to perform laparoscopy with surgical excision of discovered implants before offering other treatments can be discussed with each patient. If the patient is young, it is not unreasonable to discuss expectant management or SO/IUI as a first line therapy. If the patient is older and nearing 35, a more aggressive plan such as superovulation/IUI or IVF with or without pre-IVF ovulation suppression should be discussed with her.

For women with suspected stage III/IV endometriosis, IVF is recommended. If surgery is performed and the initial surgery does not restore fertility, IVF with or without pre-ART ovulation suppression is an effective alternative compared with repeat surgery, although there is currently insufficient evidence to assess the benefit of surgery in addition to IVF on the outcomes of pregnancy.[3]

REFERENCES

1. Olive DL, Pritts EA. Treatment of endometriosis. N Engl J Med 2001;345(4): 266–75.
2. Verkauf BS. Incidence, symptoms, and signs of endometriosis in fertile and infertile women. J Fla Med Assoc 1987;74(9):671–5.
3. The Practice Committee of the American Society for Reproductive Medicine. Endometriosis and infertility: a committee opinion. Fertil Steril 2012;98(3):591–8.
4. Hughes EG, Fedorkow DM, Collins JA. A quantitative overview of controlled trials in endometriosis-associated infertility. Fertil Steril 1993;59(5):963–70.
5. Akande VA, Hunt LP, Cahill DJ, et al. Differences in time to natural conception between women with unexplained infertility and infertile women with minor endometriosis. Hum Reprod 2004;19(1):96–103.
6. Brosens I. Endometriosis and the outcome of in vitro fertilization. Fertil Steril 2004; 81(5):1198–200.
7. Olivennes F. Resultats des FIV en cas d'endometriose. [Results of IVF in women with endometriosis]. J Gynecol Obstet Biol Reprod (Paris) 2003;32(8 Pt 2):S45–7.
8. Giudice LC, Kao LC. Endometriosis. Lancet 2004;364(9447):1789–99.
9. Olive DL, Schwartz LB. Endometriosis. N Engl J Med 1993;328(24):1759–69.
10. Sampson JA. Metastatic or embolic endometriosis, due to the menstrual dissemination of endometrial tissue into the venous circulation. Am J Pathol 1927;3(2): 93–110.43.
11. Halme J, Hammond MG, Hulka JF, et al. Retrograde menstruation in healthy women and in patients with endometriosis. Obstet Gynecol 1984;64(2):151–4.
12. D'Hooghe TM. Clinical relevance of the baboon as a model for the study of endometriosis. Fertil Steril 1997;68(4):613–25.
13. Nunley WC Jr, Kitchin JD 3rd. Congenital atresia of the uterine cervix with pelvic endometriosis. Arch Surg 1980;115(6):757–8.
14. Ferguson BR, Bennington JL, Haber SL. Histochemistry of mucosubstances and histology of mixed mullerian pelvic lymph node glandular inclusions. Evidence for histogenesis by mullerian metaplasia of coelomic epithelium. Obstet Gynecol 1969;33(5):617–25.
15. Steele RW, Dmowski WP, Marmer DJ. Immunologic aspects of human endometriosis. Am J Reprod Immunol 1984;6(1):33–6.
16. Oosterlynck DJ, Cornillie FJ, Waer M, et al. Women with endometriosis show a defect in natural killer activity resulting in a decreased cytotoxicity to autologous endometrium. Fertil Steril 1991;56(1):45–51.
17. Harada T, Iwabe T, Terakawa N. Role of cytokines in endometriosis. Fertil Steril 2001;76(1):1–10.

18. Lebovic DI, Mueller MD, Taylor RN. Immunobiology of endometriosis. Fertil Steril 2001;75(1):1–10.
19. Witz CA. Interleukin-6: another piece of the endometriosis-cytokine puzzle. Fertil Steril 2000;73(2):212–4.
20. Chan RW, Schwab KE, Gargett CE. Clonogenicity of human endometrial epithelial and stromal cells. Biol Reprod 2004;70(6):1738–50.
21. Du H, Taylor HS. Contribution of bone marrow-derived stem cells to endometrium and endometriosis. Stem Cells 2007;25(8):2082–6.
22. Taylor HS. Endometrial cells derived from donor stem cells in bone marrow transplant recipients. JAMA 2004;292(1):81–5.
23. Simpson JL, Elias S, Malinak LR, et al. Heritable aspects of endometriosis. I. Genetic studies. Am J Obstet Gynecol 1980;137(3):327–31.
24. Hadfield RM, Mardon HJ, Barlow DH, et al. Endometriosis in monozygotic twins. Fertil Steril 1997;68(5):941–2.
25. Hadfield RM, Yudkin PL, Coe CL, et al. Risk factors for endometriosis in the rhesus monkey (Macaca mulatta): a case-control study. Hum Reprod Update 1997; 3(2):109–15.
26. Bedaiwy MA, Falcone T, Mascha EJ, et al. Genetic polymorphism in the fibrinolytic system and endometriosis. Obstet Gynecol 2006;108(1):162–8.
27. Taylor HS, Bagot C, Kardana A, et al. HOX gene expression is altered in the endometrium of women with endometriosis. Hum Reprod 1999;14(5):1328–31.
28. Zanatta A, Rocha AM, Carvalho FM, et al. The role of the Hoxa10/HOXA10 gene in the etiology of endometriosis and its related infertility: a review. J Assist Reprod Genet 2010;27(12):701–10.
29. Lee B, Du H, Taylor HS. Experimental murine endometriosis induces DNA methylation and altered gene expression in eutopic endometrium. Biol Reprod 2009; 80(1):79–85.
30. Kim JJ, Taylor HS, Lu Z, et al. Altered expression of HOXA10 in endometriosis: potential role in decidualization. Mol Hum Reprod 2007;13(5):323–32.
31. Dinulescu DM, Ince TA, Quade BJ, et al. Role of K-ras and Pten in the development of mouse models of endometriosis and endometrioid ovarian cancer. Nat Med 2005;11(1):63–70.
32. Grechukhina O, Petracco R, Popkhadze S, et al. A polymorphism in a let-7 microRNA binding site of KRAS in women with endometriosis. EMBO Mol Med 2012; 4(3):206–17.
33. Holoch KJ, Lessey BA. Endometriosis and infertility. Clin Obstet Gynecol 2010; 53(2):429–38.
34. D'Hooghe TM, Debrock S, Hill JA, et al. Endometriosis and subfertility: is the relationship resolved? Semin Reprod Med 2003;21(2):243–54.
35. Oral E, Arici A, Olive DL, et al. Peritoneal fluid from women with moderate or severe endometriosis inhibits sperm motility: the role of seminal fluid components. Fertil Steril 1996;66(5):787–92.
36. Morcos RN, Gibbons WE, Findley WE. Effect of peritoneal fluid on in vitro cleavage of 2-cell mouse embryos: possible role in infertility associated with endometriosis. Fertil Steril 1985;44(5):678–83.
37. Ota H, Igarashi S, Sato N, et al. Involvement of catalase in the endometrium of patients with endometriosis and adenomyosis. Fertil Steril 2002;78(4): 804–9.
38. Ota H, Igarashi S, Kato N, et al. Aberrant expression of glutathione peroxidase in eutopic and ectopic endometrium in endometriosis and adenomyosis. Fertil Steril 2000;74(2):313–8.

39. Santamaria X, Massasa EE, Taylor HS. Migration of cells from experimental endo-metriosis to the uterine endometrium. Endocrinology 2012. [Epub ahead of print].

40. Hou X, Tan Y, Li M, et al. Canonical Wnt signaling is critical to estrogen-mediated uterine growth. Mol Endocrinol 2004;18(12):3035–49.

41. Kao LC, Germeyer A, Tulac S, et al. Expression profiling of endometrium from women with endometriosis reveals candidate genes for disease-based implanta-tion failure and infertility. Endocrinology 2003;144(7):2870–81.

42. Mohamed OA, Jonnaert M, Labelle-Dumais C, et al. Uterine Wnt/beta-catenin signaling is required for implantation. Proc Natl Acad Sci U S A 2005;102(24): 8579–84.

43. Liu Y, Kodithuwakku SP, Ng PY, et al. Excessive ovarian stimulation up-regulates the Wnt-signaling molecule DKK1 in human endometrium and may affect implan-tation: an in vitro co-culture study. Hum Reprod 2010;25(2):479–90.

44. Zeitoun KM, Bulun SE. Aromatase: a key molecule in the pathophysiology of endometriosis and a therapeutic target. Fertil Steril 1999;72(6):961–9.

45. Mote PA, Balleine RL, McGowan EM, et al. Colocalization of progesterone recep-tors A and B by dual immunofluorescent histochemistry in human endometrium during the menstrual cycle. J Clin Endocrinol Metab 1999;84(8):2963–71.

46. Lessey BA, Ilesanmi AO, Castelbaum AJ, et al. Characterization of the functional progesterone receptor in an endometrial adenocarcinoma cell line (Ishikawa): progesterone-induced expression of the alpha1 integrin. J Steroid Biochem Mol Biol 1996;59(1):31–9.

47. Lessey BA, Yeh I, Castelbaum AJ, et al. Endometrial progesterone receptors and markers of uterine receptivity in the window of implantation. Fertil Steril 1996; 65(3):477–83.

48. Osteen KG, Keller NR, Feltus FA, et al. Paracrine regulation of matrix metallopro-teinase expression in the normal human endometrium. Gynecol Obstet Invest 1999;48(Suppl 1):2–13.

49. Lessey BA, Castelbaum AJ, Sawin SW, et al. Aberrant integrin expression in the endometrium of women with endometriosis. J Clin Endocrinol Metab 1994;79(2): 643–9.

50. Ozkan S, Murk W, Arici A. Endometriosis and infertility: epidemiology and evidence-based treatments. Ann N Y Acad Sci 2008;1127:92–100.

51. Taylor HS, Osteen KG, Bruner-Tran KL, et al. Novel therapies targeting endome-triosis. Reprod Sci 2011;18(9):814–23.

52. Petracco RG, Kong A, Grechukhina O, et al. Global gene expression profiling of proliferative phase endometrium reveals distinct functional subdivisions. Reprod Sci 2012;19(10):1138–45.

53. Marcoux S, Maheux R, Berube S. Laparoscopic surgery in infertile women with minimal or mild endometriosis. Canadian Collaborative Group on Endometriosis. N Engl J Med 1997;337(4):217–22.

54. Berube S, Marcoux S, Langevin M, et al. Fecundity of infertile women with minimal or mild endometriosis and women with unexplained infertility. The Canadian Collaborative Group on Endometriosis. Fertil Steril 1998;69(6):1034–41.

55. Zeitoun K, Takayama K, Sasano H, et al. Deficient 17beta-hydroxysteroid dehy-drogenase type 2 expression in endometriosis: failure to metabolize 17beta-estradiol. J Clin Endocrinol Metab 1998;83(12):4474–80.

56. Hughes E, Brown J, Collins JJ, et al. Ovulation suppression for endometriosis. Cochrane Database Syst Rev 2007;(3):CD000155.

57. Rocha AL, Reis FM, Petraglia F. New trends for the medical treatment of endome-triosis. Expert Opin Investig Drugs 2012;21(7):905–19.

58. Guo YH, Lu N, Zhang Y, et al. Comparative study on the pregnancy outcomes of in vitro fertilization-embryo transfer between long-acting gonadotropin-releasing hormone agonist combined with transvaginal ultrasound-guided cyst aspiration and long-acting gonadotropin-releasing hormone agonist alone. Contemp Clin Trials 2012;33(6):1206–10.
59. Ozkan S, Arici A. Advances in treatment options of endometriosis. Gynecol Obstet Invest 2009;67(2):81–91.
60. Surrey ES, Voigt B, Fournet N, et al. Prolonged gonadotropin-releasing hormone agonist treatment of symptomatic endometriosis: the role of cyclic sodium etidronate and low-dose norethindrone "add-back" therapy. Fertil Steril 1995;63(4):747–55.
61. Surrey ES, Silverberg KM, Surrey MW, et al. Effect of prolonged gonadotropin-releasing hormone agonist therapy on the outcome of in vitro fertilization-embryo transfer in patients with endometriosis. Fertil Steril 2002;78(4):699–704.
62. Olivennes F, Feldberg D, Liu HC, et al. Endometriosis: a stage by stage analysis–the role of in vitro fertilization. Fertil Steril 1995;64(2):392–8.
63. Sallam HN, Garcia-Velasco JA, Dias S, et al. Long-term pituitary down-regulation before in vitro fertilization (IVF) for women with endometriosis. Cochrane Database Syst Rev 2006;(1):CD004635.
64. de Ziegler D, Gayet V, Aubriot FX, et al. Use of oral contraceptives in women with endometriosis before assisted reproduction treatment improves outcomes. Fertil Steril 2010;94(7):2796–9.
65. Benschop L, Farquhar C, van der Poel N, et al. Interventions for women with endometrioma prior to assisted reproductive technology. Cochrane Database Syst Rev 2010;(11):CD008571.
66. Kennedy S, Bergqvist A, Chapron C, et al. ESHRE guideline for the diagnosis and treatment of endometriosis. Hum Reprod 2005;20(10):2698–704.
67. Busacca M, Fedele L, Bianchi S, et al. Surgical treatment of recurrent endometriosis: laparotomy versus laparoscopy. Hum Reprod 1998;13(8):2271–4.
68. Parazzini F. Ablation of lesions or no treatment in minimal-mild endometriosis in infertile women: a randomized trial. Gruppo Italiano per lo Studio dell'Endometriosi. Hum Reprod 1999;14(5):1332–4.
69. Jacobson TZ, Barlow DH, Koninckx PR, et al. Laparoscopic surgery for subfertility associated with endometriosis. Cochrane Database Syst Rev 2002;(4):CD001398.
70. Jacobson TZ, Duffy JM, Barlow D, et al. Laparoscopic surgery for subfertility associated with endometriosis. Cochrane Database Syst Rev 2010;(1):CD001398.
71. Hart RJ, Hickey M, Maouris P, et al. Excisional surgery versus ablative surgery for ovarian endometriomata. Cochrane Database Syst Rev 2008;(2):CD004992.
72. Audebert A, Descamps P, Marret H, et al. Pre or post-operative medical treatment with nafarelin in stage III-IV endometriosis: a French multicenter study. Eur J Obstet Gynecol Reprod Biol 1998;79(2):145–8.
73. Muzii L, Marana R, Caruana P, et al. The impact of preoperative gonadotropin-releasing hormone agonist treatment on laparoscopic excision of ovarian endometriotic cysts. Fertil Steril 1996;65(6):1235–7.
74. Furness S, Roberts H, Marjoribanks J, et al. Hormone therapy in postmenopausal women and risk of endometrial hyperplasia. Cochrane Database Syst Rev 2009;(2):CD000402.
75. Fedele L, Bianchi S, Marchini M, et al. Superovulation with human menopausal gonadotropins in the treatment of infertility associated with minimal or mild endometriosis: a controlled randomized study. Fertil Steril 1992;58(1):28–31.

76. Guzick DS. Randomized controlled trial of superovulation and insemination for infertility associated with minimal or mild endometriosis. J Womens Health 1997;6(4):489–90.
77. Senapati S, Barnhart K. Managing endometriosis-associated infertility. Clin Obstet Gynecol 2011;54(4):720–6.
78. Tummon IS, Asher LJ, Martin JS, et al. Randomized controlled trial of superovulation and insemination for infertility associated with minimal or mild endometriosis. Fertil Steril 1997;68(1):8–12.
79. Deaton JL, Gibson M, Blackmer KM, et al. A randomized, controlled trial of clomiphene citrate and intrauterine insemination in couples with unexplained infertility or surgically corrected endometriosis. Fertil Steril 1990;54(6):1083–8.
80. Abu Hashim H, El Rakhawy M, Abd Elaal I. Randomized comparison of superovulation with letrozole vs. clomiphene citrate in an IUI program for women with recently surgically treated minimal to mild endometriosis. Acta Obstet Gynecol Scand 2012;91(3):338–45.
81. Dmowski WP, Pry M, Ding J, et al. Cycle-specific and cumulative fecundity in patients with endometriosis who are undergoing controlled ovarian hyperstimulation-intrauterine insemination or in vitro fertilization-embryo transfer. Fertil Steril 2002;78(4):750–6.
82. Assisted reproductive technology in the United States: 2010 results generated from the American Society for Reproductive Medicine/Society for Assisted Reproduction registry [database on the Internet]. 2012.
83. Opoien HK, Fedorcsak P, Omland AK, et al. In vitro fertilization is a successful treatment in endometriosis-associated infertility. Fertil Steril 2012;97(4):912–8.
84. Bukulmez O, Yarali H, Gurgan T. The presence and extent of endometriosis do not effect clinical pregnancy and implantation rates in patients undergoing intracytoplasmic sperm injection. Eur J Obstet Gynecol Reprod Biol 2001;96(1):102–7.
85. Guo SW. Epigenetics of endometriosis. Mol Hum Reprod 2009;15(10):587–607.

Tubal Factor Infertility
Diagnosis and Management in the Era of Assisted Reproductive Technology

Erica C. Dun, MD, MPH[a], Ceana H. Nezhat, MD[a,b,c],*

KEYWORDS

- Tubal factor infertility • In vitro fertilization • Microsurgery • Tubal occlusion

KEY POINTS

- Tubal factor infertility is the most common cause of female infertility.
- The diagnosis of tubal factor infertility can be established by a combination of clinical suspicion based on patient history and confirmed with diagnostic tests.
- Depending on the patient's age, location, and severity of tubal disease, tubal microsurgery or more commonly in vitro fertilization with its improving success rates are the recommended treatment options.

INFERTILITY IS A GROWING CONCERN

Approximately 85% to 90% of healthy young couples conceive within 1 year of trying, and most conceive within 6 months.[1] However, 10% to 15% of couples have difficulty conceiving and experience infertility or subfertility, which is defined as 1 year of unprotected intercourse without conception.[2] Although overall rates of infertility have remained stable during the last 30 years in the United States the overall birth and fertility rates are declining because of several social and cultural trends: women achieving advanced education and careers, delaying marriage for men and women, delaying childbearing, more frequent divorce, and reliable contraception and family planning. Comparatively, the first US census in 1790 indicated that the crude birth rate was 55 per 1000 of the total population. During the postwar "baby boom" of

Conflicts of interest: Dr Erica Dun declares no conflicts of interest. Dr Ceana Nezhat is a consultant for Conceptus, Hologic, Lumenis, Intuitive Surgical, and Karl Storz; medical advisor for Plasma Surgical; and on the scientific advisory board for SurgiQuest.
Financial support: No financial support was received to write this article.
[a] Atlanta Center for Minimally Invasive Surgery and Reproductive Medicine, 5555 Peachtree Dunwoody Road, Suite 276, Atlanta, GA 30342, USA; [b] Emory University, Atlanta, GA, USA; [c] Stanford University, CA, USA
* Corresponding author.
E-mail address: Ceana@Nezhat.com

the 1950s, the fertility rate (births per 1000 women aged 15–44) peaked at 106.2 per 1000. The most recent statistics from the Centers for Disease Control and Prevention report a falling fertility rate of 66.7 per 1000 in 2009. Interestingly, although the birth rates are declining for women age 15 to 39 years, the birth rates continue to rise for women 40 to 44 years.[3]

Because of societal trends, female infertility is a growing and important issue. Much attention in the past 30 years has been focused on understanding the physiology of reproductive aging and finding treatments for all causes of infertility.

Among infertile couples, male infertility accounts for approximately 35% and female infertility approximately 65% (**Fig. 1**). The causes of male infertility arise from four major etiologies: (1) hypothalamic-pituitary disorders (1%–2%); (2) primary gonadal disorders (30%–40%); (3) disorders of sperm transport (10%–20%); and (4) idiopathic (40%–50%). Most male factor infertility is still idiopathic, reflecting a poor understanding of the mechanisms that govern testicular and sperm function. However, female infertility represents approximately 65% of the overall causes for the infertile couple. The components of female reproductive process can be divided into the following anatomic components. Dysfunction may occur at any of these steps to cause infertility: (1) the ovaries need to ovulate a mature oocyte on a regular basis (ovarian factor); (2) the cervix needs to capture and transport sperm into the uterus and fallopian tubes (cervical factor); (3) the uterus needs to allow the embryo to implant and support normal growth and development (uterine factor); and (4) the fallopian tubes need to capture the ovulated ova and transport sperm and embryo (tubal factor).

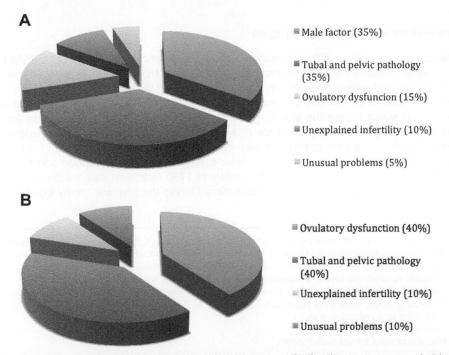

A

■ Male factor (35%)

■ Tubal and pelvic pathology (35%)

▪ Ovulatory dysfuncion (15%)

▪ Unexplained infertility (10%)

▪ Unusual problems (5%)

B

▪ Ovulatory dysfunction (40%)

■ Tubal and pelvic pathology (40%)

▪ Unexplained infertility (10%)

■ Unusual problems (10%)

Fig. 1. (*A*) Causes of infertility among couples. (*B*) Causes of infertility in younger and older women. (*Data from* Miller JH, Weinberg RK, Canino NL, et al. The pattern of infertility diagnoses in women of advanced reproductive age. Am J Obstet Gynecol 1999;181:952–7.)

Dysfunction caused by the last component of the female reproductive pathway, tubal factor infertility, is the most common cause of female infertility and is discussed in this article.

CAUSES OF TUBAL FACTOR INFERTILITY

Tubal factor infertility due to occlusion and peritoneal pathology causing adhesions is the most common cause of female infertility and diagnosed in approximately 30% to 35% of younger and older infertile women.[4] The most prevalent cause of tubal factor infertility is pelvic inflammatory disease (PID) and acute salpingitis. *Chlamydia trachomatis*, *Neisseria gonorrhea*, and anaerobic organisms are the most common organisms that infect the lower genital tract and cause PID. In classic studies of women diagnosed with PID, the risk of infertility increased with the number and severity of pelvic infections. The incidence of infertility is 10% to 12% after one episode, 23% to 35% after two episodes, and 54% to 75% after three episodes.[5,6] Tubal damage from PID causes inflammation and long-term tubal changes, such as fimbrial agglutination, fimbrial phimosis, tubal obstruction, hydrosalpinx, and nodular thickening of the muscularis layer of the isthmic portion of the fallopian tube called salpingitis isthmica nodosa. The risk of ectopic pregnancy can increase sixfold to sevenfold after an episode of PID.[7]

Endometriosis is a common and chronic inflammatory disorder affecting 10% to 16% of reproductive-aged women.[8] Among women with infertility, pelvic pain, or both, it is present in 35% to 50%.[9] Although the pathophysiology of endometriosis is not completely understood, the most accepted theory is retrograde menstruation of debris from the uterus through the fallopian tubes that attach to the peritoneal surfaces. Women who develop endometriosis are unable to clear the disseminated endometrial cells, and may have altered humoral and cellular immune systems. Chronic inflammation from the reactive cytokines and chemokines produced by the ectopic endometrium results in scarring similar to that observed in PID. The long-term consequence of the inflammation is often distal tubal adhesive disease and occlusion. Among women with tubal factor infertility, endometriosis accounts for 7% to 14% **(Fig. 2)**.[10]

Although uncommon in the United States, worldwide tuberculosis is reported to infect 9.4 million new people each year.[11] Among patients with pulmonary tuberculosis, the incidence of pelvic tuberculosis is between 10% and 20%.[12] The most common clinical symptoms of pelvic tuberculosis are pelvic pain, general malaise, menstrual irregularity, and infertility. Both fallopian tubes usually develop salpingitis,

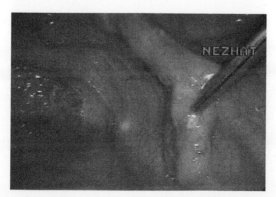

Fig. 2. Laparoscopy of a patient with endometriosis present on the fimbriae of the fallopian tube.

which in later stages resembles PID. Large, caseous pyosalpinges are characteristic of tuberculosis infection, but the pyosalpinges may also contain the exudate of a secondary infection with other urogenital organisms. Before effective multiregimen antibiotics, the treatment of pelvic tuberculosis was surgical, but was frequently complicated by fistula formation and persistent draining sinuses. Currently, surgery is reserved for women who have failed medical therapy and either have a persistent adnexal mass after 4 to 6 months of antituberculosis antibiotic therapy or unrelieved pelvic pain while on medical therapy.[13]

Other causes of tubal factor infertility include scarring from abdominal and pelvic surgeries. Ruptured appendix increases the risk of tubal infertility (relative risk = 4.8; 95% confidence interval, 1.5–14.9).[14] Inflammatory bowel disease was once thought to decrease fertility, but population-based studies of women with Crohn disease reported infertility rates between 5% and 14%, which are similar to the general population.[15,16] Women with ulcerative colitis have similar rates of fertility.[17] However, after surgery for both inflammatory bowel diseases, fertility rates decreased possibly because of surgery in the pelvis and subsequent adhesions and damage to the reproductive organs.[18]

Myomas near the tubal ostium can occlude the cornua and interstitial portion of the fallopian tube, causing or creating the appearance of proximal fallopian tube blockage. Depending on the degree of anatomic distortion, myomectomy can be complicated because removal of the fibroid may not restore fallopian tube patency. Meticulous surgical repair of the cornual with intraoperative chromopertubation can determine if the tube is patent at the end of the procedure (**Fig. 3**).

Bilateral tubal ligation is an iatrogenic cause of tubal occlusion. The traditional post-partum tubal ligation consists of ligating a knuckle at the midisthmic portion of the fallopian tube. Laparoscopic tubal ligation methods include monopolar and bipolar cautery, Hulka Clips, Fallope Rings, and Filshie Clips. Essure and Adiana are permanent hysteroscopic methods of proximal tubal occlusion. The microinsert is placed into the interstitium, scarring the fallopian tube, and occluding the proximal portions of the tubes over 3 months. A hysterosalpingogram (HSG) is performed after the 3 months to document occlusion.

PATIENT HISTORY

The patient's medical history can provide valuable information to assess the risk for tubal disease. A history of the risk factors, such as PID, septic abortion, ruptured

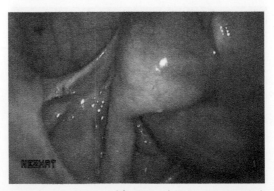

Fig. 3. Laparoscopy revealing a uterus with cornual myoma compressing the tubal ostium and causing proximal tube occlusion.

appendix, tubal surgery, or ectopic pregnancy is highly suggestive of tubal damage and dysfunction. Chronic medical conditions including endometriosis, or multiple abdominal and pelvic surgeries increase the amount of inflammation and scarring in and around the fallopian tubes and ovaries. A history of permanent sterilization by tubal ligation is a clear indicator of tubal occlusion. Gathering a thorough review of symptoms is essential to elicit symptoms of pelvic and abdominal pain, dyschezia, and dyspareunia.

PHYSICAL EXAMINATION

Evaluation of the infertile female patient should include a complete physical examination. Weight and body mass index should be noted. Thyroid enlargement, tenderness or nodularity, breast secretions, signs of androgen excess, such as facial and body hair and acne, or insulin resistance suggest some common endocrine causes of infertility (ie, thyroid dysfunction, hyperprolactinemia, and polycystic ovarian syndrome). In women with infertility and history of risk factors for tubal disease, the abdominal and pelvic examination is particularly important and assists in the diagnosis. Pelvic or abdominal tenderness, organ enlargement or masses on examination, vaginal or cervical abnormalities, secretions, and abnormal discharge help to differentiate anatomic abnormalities, neoplasia, or infection. A Pap smear and cervical cultures should be performed during the pelvic examination. The bimanual examination can provide information regarding uterine contour irregularity. Lack of uterine mobility indicates potential scarring from previous surgeries or disease processes. A rectovaginal examination should be performed to diagnose tenderness, nodularity, or masses in the adnexa or cul-de-sac suggestive of endometriosis.

IMAGING AND ADDITIONAL TESTING TO DIAGNOSE TUBAL FACTOR INFERTILITY
Laparoscopy and Chromopertubation

Laparoscopy with chromopertubation is considered the definitive test for evaluating tubal disease. Laparoscopy is performed under general anesthesia, and is often combined with chromopertubation (injection of a dilute blue dye though a cannula that passes through the cervix into the uterus, allowing the dye to enter the uterine cavity and fallopian tubes) to evaluate tubal patency and hysteroscopy to evaluate the interior of the uterus. Laparoscopy provides a panoramic view of the abdomen and pelvis and allows surgeons to diagnose and treat various pathologies, such as distal tubal occlusive disease, endometriosis, and adnexal and pelvic adhesions. Intraoperative chromopertubation is a better test for diagnosing tubal patency than HSG because there is less observer variability. However, cornual spasms, which are uterine contractions that transiently close the interstitial segment, can confound the results if the dye is injected too quickly. The cornual spasm causes the false appearance of proximal tube occlusion. Nevertheless, information obtained from laparoscopies tends to be more accurate than HSG, and is a better indicator of future fertility (**Fig. 4**).[19]

Hysterosalpingography

HSG is an outpatient radiographic procedure that examines fallopian tube patency. It is ideally performed 2 to 5 days immediately after the end of menses to minimize the interference from blood clot and menstrual debris, to prevent the chance that the procedure may be performed after conception, and to minimize the risk of infection. C trachomatis has been cultured in up to 3.4% of women scheduled to undergo an HSG.[20] Postprocedure PID is uncommon, occurring in less than 1.4% of women

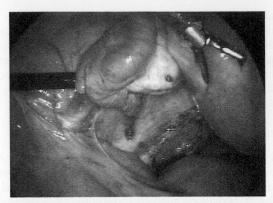

Fig. 4. Laparoscopy with chromopertubation demonstrating a patent fallopian tube with dilute methylene blue dye emanating from the fimbriae.

undergoing an HSG. Women with dilated fallopian tubes had a significantly higher risk (11%) of postprocedure PID.[21] However, it is a potentially devastating postprocedure complication, especially in a group of women undergoing infertility evaluation. Consequently, because of the risk of lower genital tract infection at the time of the procedure, doxycycline, 100 mg twice a day for 5 days, beginning 1 to 2 days before the procedure is recommended[22] to prevent postprocedure PID. If a woman has had an episode of PID, the HSG should be delayed at least several weeks after the infection has resolved.

The HSG procedure is standard and preprocedure preparation is simple and involves the doxycycline regimen outlined previously and ibuprofen 30 to 60 minutes before the procedure to minimize discomfort during the procedure. The patient is in a supine position on a fluoroscopy-read table and a metal "acorn" cannula or a balloon catheter is placed into the cervix and lower segment of the uterus. Water-soluble or oil-soluble contrast media is injected into the cannula or catheter, which directs the contrast media into the uterine cavity and fallopian tubes. Fluoroscopy guides the imaging over the patient's pelvis. Three basic films are required for documenting an adequate study: (1) a scout film of the lower abdomen and pelvis, (2) a film to document the uterine contours and tubal patency, and (3) a postevaluation film to detect areas of contrast loculation that may indicate peritubal adhesive disease. Additional oblique films may be needed if the uterus obscures the tubes or if the uterine cavity seems abnormal.

Although traditional laparoscopy with chromopertubation is the gold standard for investigating tubal patency, HSG has moderate sensitivity (65%) but excellent specificity (83%) in the infertile population. However, if the HSG indicates occlusion, there may be a good chance (60%) that the tubes are actually patent, and if the HSG demonstrates patency there is a little chance (5%) that the tubes are occluded.[23,24] The primary reason for the moderate sensitivity is twofold: injection of the HSG contrast material causes cornual spasm more commonly than the dilute dye used in laparoscopic chromopertubation and the interpretation of the HSG is subject to intraobserver variability.[25] Nevertheless, HSG is a valuable, less-invasive method of examining tubal patency. HSG has advantages over laparoscopy aside from being a faster, less invasive, and less expensive procedure. It can delineate the contours of the uterine cavity and the lumen of the fallopian tubes. An incidental but important finding with the use of oil-soluble contrast media is that it has been shown to increase fertility in the months immediately after the procedure in women with patent tubes.[26] The thought is the oil-soluble contrast material flushes tubal debris from the tubal lumen (**Fig. 5**).[27]

Sonohysterosalpingography

Sonohysterosalpingography (SHG) is an alternative imaging technique to the HSG. SHG is an ultrasound-based imaging modality that permits an accurate evaluation of tubal patency and uterine and ovarian pathology. Use of a sonographic contrast medium (eg, sterile saline, air, Echovist, Albunex, and Infoson) injected into the uterine cavity enhances visualization of the uterine contours and fallopian tubes. If at least one fallopian tube is patent, then fluid accumulates in the posterior cul-de-sac during the procedure. Use of three-dimensional imaging to generate coronal images and Doppler to highlight fluid movement through the fallopian tubes can further improve the diagnostic capabilities of the SHG.

There are several advantages of the SHG. It is a fast, low-cost test that can be performed in an outpatient setting without anesthesia or sedation. There is no exposure to radiation. It is better tolerated than the HSG,[28] with fewer side effects rated as moderate to severe pain, vasovagal symptoms, nausea, and vomiting. Serious postprocedure complications (eg, fever and peritonitis) occurred in only 0.95% of the procedures.[29,30] Although the sonographic images are inferior to fluoroscopy, SHG is more sensitive and specific than the HSG when evaluating tubal patency. In fact, a meta-analysis comparing the accuracy of HSG, SHG, and laparoscopy found that SHG was superior to HSG and comparable with laparoscopic chromopertubation to demonstrate tubal patency (**Fig. 6**).[31]

Chlamydia serology

Chlamydia antibody tests (CAT) are a simple and noninvasive method of assessing tubal disease. They are blood tests that can detect previous infection with *C trachomatis*, an obligate intracellular bacteria that causes PID and subsequent fallopian tube injury and dysfunction.[32] Four commercial assay methods for detecting *Chlamydia* are currently available: (1) immunofluorescence, (2) microimmunofluorescence, (3) enzyme-linked immunosorbent assay, and (4) immunoperoxidase. The microimmunofluorescence test is the most specific for *C trachomatis*, detecting its type-specific

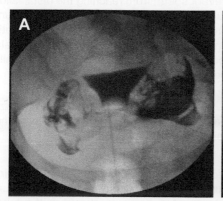
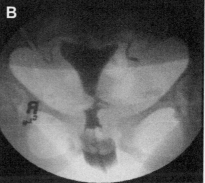

Fig. 5. (*A*) Normal HSG with patent fallopian tubes. The contrast material has moved through both fallopian tubes and spilled into the cul-de-sac, indicating bilateral tubal patency. (*B*) Abnormal HSG showing bilateral distal tubal occlusion. The contrast material fills the uterine cavity and flows through most of the fallopian tubes, but there is no spill of the contrast material into the cul-de-sac, indicating a distal tubal occlusion.

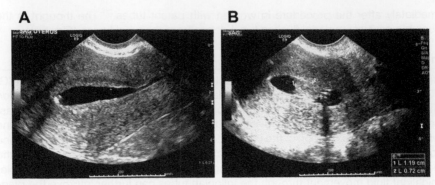

Fig. 6. (*A*) A normal SHG. The uterine cavity is distended, and the endometrium is smooth and without intracavitary defects. The myometrium is homogeneous. (*B*) A SHG demonstrating an intracavitary myoma.

immunoglobulin G antibodies. Other methods are not as specific, and do not distinguish between *C trachomatis* and the antibodies of other *Chlamydia* species, *Chlamydia pneumonia* and *Chlamydia psittaci*. Mol and colleagues[33] performed meta-analysis comparing CAT with HSG for the diagnosis of tubal occlusion using laparoscopic chromopertubation as the standard. The microimmunofluorescence test has a sensitivity less than 75%, but a specificity greater than 75%. Several limitations cloud the use of this test, including false-positive results caused by cross-reactivity with some gram-negative bacterial lipopolysaccharides and false-negative results in women with mild *Chlamydia* infections.[32] Thus, the role for CAT in the evaluation of infertile women has not been clearly defined. These serologic tests may be most suitable as a screening test to classify women into low- or high-risk groups for tubal disease warranting further investigation with more invasive tests, such as HSG, SHG, or laparoscopy.

MANAGEMENT OF TUBAL FACTOR INFERTILITY

Fallopian tube disease can roughly be divided into proximal tube and distal tube obstruction. Proximal tubal obstructions prevent sperm from reaching the distal fallopian tube where fertilization normally occurs. Distal tubal occlusion prevents ovum capture from the ovary, but can exhibit a range of disease from mild (fimbrial agglutination); moderate (varying degrees of fimbrial phimosis); and severe (complete obstruction). Damage to internal tubal mucosal structures cannot be detected easily and normal tubal function is difficult to assess.

Tubal Surgery

After diagnostic testing has indicated tubal occlusion, interventional radiology and microsurgical techniques can restore fallopian tube anatomy and function.

Proximal tubal occlusion

Proximal tubal blockage accounts for 10% to 24% of tubal disease.[34] Selective salpingography is a radiographic procedure similar to HSG in which the fallopian tube is directly opacified under fluoroscopic guidance. A catheter is placed in the tubal ostium, and a radiopaque dye is injected into the fallopian tube to determine patency. The procedure is usually performed by interventional radiologists and has been used to differentiate tubal spasm from true tubal obstruction. The advantage of this procedure is that if an obstruction is identified, a subsequent fallopian tube recanalization can be performed during which a smaller catheter is placed to clear the obstruction. The recanalization procedure is simple and successfully completed in 71% to 92% of cases.[35] Recanalization is possible but less successful in women who have occluded tubes after surgical anastomosis for reversal of a tubal ligation. Reported success rates per fallopian tube are related to amount of postoperative scarring and range from 44% to 77%.[36] Of the women who had successful fallopian tube recanalization, the average pregnancy rate was 30%.[37–40] Complications from the procedure are rare and include perforation in 3% to 11% of cases without clinical sequelae[34] and an ectopic pregnancy rate of 3%, which is comparable with the general population.[41] If the obstruction is not resolved by tubal cannulation, then in vitro fertilization (IVF) is preferred to proximal tube resection and microsurgical proximal tube anastomosis. Microsurgical proximal tube anastomosis has been largely relegated to historic surgical interest, because it is associated with very low success rates and risk of cornual rupture in pregnancy. It should only be considered if IVF is not an option for the patient.

Distal tubal occlusion

Distal tubal occlusion accounts for most tubal occlusion and infertility. Microsurgery can treat most cases depending on the degree of occlusion. A successful outcome with tubal surgery is associated with no more than limited filmy adnexal adhesions; mildly dilated tubes (<3 cm in diameter) with thin and pliable walls; and a lush endosalpinx with preservation of the mucosal folds.[42] Salpingostomy involves creating an opening in a completely obstructed tube, and historically was performed at laparotomy with microscopic assistance. More recently, laparoscopic salpingostomy has been performed with equivalent results.[43] Unfortunately, salpingostomy yields low long-term pregnancy rates of approximately 20% to 30% 1 to 2 years after surgery[43,44]; rates vary considerably depending on the extent of tubal damage and other clinical factors. Ectopic pregnancy rates after salpingostomy range from 4% to 25%.[44]

Varying degrees of fimbrial disease can be laparoscopically treated with fimbroplasty and fimbriolysis. Fimbriolysis refers to the separation of adherent fimbria. Fimbrioplasty describes the correction of phimotic but patent fimbria. Surgical success is inversely related to the severity of disease. For mild forms of distal tubal occlusion, pregnancy rates have been reported up to 60%,[45] but success rates are lower at 10% to 35% for women with severe tubal disease.[46,47] Most of the pregnancies occur within the first 2 years after surgical treatment of distal tubal disease. There is almost no role for surgical intervention in patients with proximal and distal disease because live birth rates are invariably lower than 10%.[45]

Hydrosalpinges

Distal tubal occlusion from salpingitis or extrinsic causes may lead to formation of hydrosalpinges either in one or both fallopian tubes. Numerous studies have shown that hydrosalpinges have a negative effect on pregnancy and IVF success rates. In a large meta-analysis of retrospective cases, women with hydrosalpinx had half the pregnancy, implantation, and delivery rates, and up to twice the incidence of spontaneous abortions after IVF and embryo transfer (IVF-ET).[48,49] Although the hydrosalpingeal fluid does not have direct toxic effects on the human embryos,[50,51] leakage of the fluid into the uterine cavity may compromise implantation through decreasing endometrial receptivity[52,53] and mechanically washing the blastocyst from the endometrial surface.[54] Treatment options for hydrosalpinges include drainage, neosalpingostomy, salpingectomy, and proximal tubal occlusion.

The least invasive of these options is transvaginal needle aspiration of a hydrosalpinx under ultrasound guidance before an IVF-ET cycle or at the time of oocyte retrieval. Therapeutic aspirations of hydrosalpinges have been reported[55,56]; however, there is often rapid reaccumulation of fluid. Nonrandomized study results were conflicting and conclusions weak.[55,57] One randomized controlled trial (RCT) reported improved pregnancy outcomes,[58] but this study was underpowered, leaving the need for more studies to assess the benefits and outcomes of hydrosalpinx aspiration. Laparoscopic neosalpingostomy for draining hydrosalpinges before IVF-ET theoretically should improve pregnancy rates, but there are no confirmatory studies to date.[59]

Randomized clinical trials comparing pregnancy rates and outcomes with IVF in women with and without prior laparoscopic salpingectomy have consistently reported that salpingectomy restores pregnancy rates and live birth rates to those similar to women without hydrosalpinx.[60–62] The multicenter, prospective RCT by Strandell and colleagues[60] found significantly increased pregnancy and live birth rates of 37% and 29%, respectively, in the salpingectomy group compared with rates of 24% and 16%, respectively, in the nonintervention group. A Cochrane analysis of the three RCTs concluded that laparoscopic salpingectomy should be considered before IVF for women with communicating hydrosalpinges.[63] Meta-analysis of two laparoscopic proximal tubal occlusion studies[62,64] also found improved odds of clinical pregnancy.[63] Thus, both salpingectomy and proximal tubal occlusion are recommended for the treatment of hydrosalpinx before IVF-ET.

Sterilization reversal

Approximately 1 million women in the United States have tubal ligations each year. Up to 7% regret the permanent sterilization, and about 1% request tubal reversal.[65] For those women who want to conceive, there are two treatment options: IVF or tubal reanastomosis. The advantages of surgical tubal reanastomosis are the chance for natural conception and lower risk for multiple gestations, but the disadvantages are the potential tubal scarring from the surgery itself, delay in attempting conception, higher risk of ectopic pregnancy, and need for future contraception.

Tubotubal reanastomosis is traditionally achieved by laparotomy after laparoscopic assessment of the fallopian tubes. If one or both fallopian tubes are judged to be repairable, then the occluded ends of the proximal and distal segments are opened and the ends are anastomosed with a fine nonreactive suture. Koh and Janik[66] reported the first case of laparoscopic tubal reanastomosis in 1992, but only laparoscopists skilled in microsurgical reanastamosis have been able to successfully replicate the procedure. More recently, more surgeons are using the da Vinci Robotic Surgical System for laparoscopic tubal reanastamosis with good results.[67,68] Women with tubal occlusion caused by tubal ligation are typically fertile and have better success rates after tubal surgery than women with tubal pathology. They also have good success rates with IVF. A preoperative HSG may be useful to assess the proximal segment of the tube. Less than 5% of fallopian tubes are irreparable. The prognosis for achieving live birth after tubal reversal depends on the patient's age, type and location of the sterilization procedure, and the final length of the repaired fallopian tubes. Better success rates are reported in younger women with no other infertility factors, and sterilization performed with rings or clips.[69] In appropriately selected candidates, overall conception rates are good (62%–83%) after microsurgical sterilization reversal.[46,70–72] The risk for ectopic pregnancy after tubal reanastomosis is up to 6%, and higher after isthmic-ampullary anastomosis than after isthmic-isthmic anastomosis.[46] Sterilization reversal after hysteroscopic placement of the microinserts Essure and Adiana is very difficult to achieve because of the placement of the coils, which scar and occlude the isthmic portions of the fallopian tubes. Sterilization reversal of this type requires tubouterine implantation in which a new opening is created through the uterine muscle and the remaining tubal segment is inserted into the uterine cavity. During the same procedure the microinserts are removed. Data on the success rate of tubal reversal after intratubal microinserts are limited. Three case reports of successful tubouterine implantation after intratubal microinserts have been described.[73,74]

Advancements in reproductive surgery with the da Vinci Surgical System

The da Vinci Robotic Surgical System developed by Intuitive Surgical (Sunnyvale, CA) pioneered one of the first integrated three-dimensional viewing systems for minimally invasive surgery. The system was approved for laparoscopic hysterectomies in 2005, but since that time has expanded to include myomectomy, complex resections of endometriosis, sacral colpopexy, and tubal reanastomosis. The high-definition video system and three-dimensional viewer have tremendously enabled surgeons to perform laparoscopic microtubal surgery with good results.

Gargiulo and Nezhat[75] reported their experience with a variety of robotic-assisted gynecologic surgeries including robotic-assisted tubal reanastomosis and tubal reconstructive surgeries citing the three-dimensional visualization of the operative field, decreased surgeon fatigue, and the seven degrees of motion provided better dexterity and surgical precision.[76–80]

Logically, using the da Vinci Surgical System for the technically challenging and microscopic procedures in reproductive surgery has been a natural progression for this surgical tool. Techniques for the robot-assisted tubal reanastomosis and other complex surgical procedures are described in recent publications.[75,81] A series comparing outcomes between women undergoing robotic-assisted tubal anastomoses and open microsurgical tubal anastomosis demonstrated that the robotically assisted laparoscopic microsurgical tubal anastomosis was feasible and cost effective with results equivalent to the traditional open approach.[82] In a series of 10 women with prior bilateral tubal ligation, 19 fallopian tubes were reanastomosed using the robotic-assisted laparoscopy technique. Chromopertubation at the end of the surgery demonstrated patency in all tubes. At 6 weeks after surgery HSGs were performed, and 17 of 19 tubes were patent. Five intrauterine pregnancies were reported.[83] The advantages of the da Vinci Surgical System are clear, and it has the potential to revolutionize the field of reproductive surgery.

In Vitro Fertilization

As assisted reproductive technologies (ART) have improved over the past few decades, almost all causes of infertility, especially tubal factor infertility, have been treated though ART techniques. In the past decade alone, the percentages of transfers that resulted in singleton live births have increased from 26% in 2000 to 35% in 2009.[84] The results of IVF-ET and tubal surgery are difficult to compare because surgery and IVF-ET have variable results depending on the surgeon and IVF clinic. One prospective RCT comparing tubal surgery to infertility with IVF-ET as first-line therapy found that the former was associated with lower costs and higher overall pregnancy rates.[85] However, a Cochrane analysis concluded that the success of tubal surgery versus IVF remains largely unknown, and in the treatment of women with tubal factor infertility, there are no RCTs comparing IVF-ET with tubal surgery.[86] When a couple is deciding between IVF-ET or tubal surgery, the advantages and disadvantages of both should be discussed. The advantages of IVF-ET are good per cycle success rates, it is less surgically invasive, and attempts at conceiving can start immediately. Disadvantages of IVF are risk of multiple gestations, ovarian hyperstimulation, and high cost. Some adverse perinatal outcomes have been associated with pregnancies conceived through IVF, such as perinatal mortality, preterm delivery, low and very low birth weight infants, intrauterine growth restriction, and congenital malformations.[87,88] Nevertheless, women who are older, women with severe tubal disease, couples with male factor infertility, and couples who may only want one or two children should be counseled toward infertility management with ART. Patient preference, religious beliefs, cost, and insurance reimbursement also play a role in management.

SUMMARY

Tubal factor infertility accounts for a large portion of female factor infertility. PID and salpingitis seem to be the most common culprits causing tubal scarring and occlusion. The diagnosis of tubal occlusion can be established by a combination of clinical suspicion based on patient history and diagnostic tests, such as HSG, SHG, and laparoscopy with chromopertubation. Depending on several patient factors, tubal microsurgery, or more commonly IVF with its improving success rates, are the recommended treatment options. Many variables need to be taken into consideration when counseling patients with tubal factor infertility about their treatment options. These factors include the age of the woman and ovarian reserve, male fertility and sperm quality, number of children desired, site and extent of fallopian tube disease, risk of ectopic pregnancy, other infertility factors, cost of the treatments, and patient preference. Nonetheless, innovative and optimistic surgical and ART treatments are now available for infertile couples.

REFERENCES

1. Gnoth C, Godehardt D, Godehardt E, et al. Time to pregnancy: results of the German prospective study and impact on the management of infertility. Hum Reprod 2003;18:1959–66.
2. Gnoth C, Godehardt E, Frank-Herrmann P, et al. Definition and prevalence of subfertility and infertility. Hum Reprod 2005;20:1144–7.
3. Martin JA, Hamilton BE, Ventura SJ, et al. Births: final data for 2009. Natl Vital Stat Rep 2011;60:1–70.
4. Miller JH, Weinberg RK, Canino NL, et al. The pattern of infertility diagnoses in women of advanced reproductive age. Am J Obstet Gynecol 1999;181:952–7.
5. Westrom L. Effect of acute pelvic inflammatory disease on fertility. Am J Obstet Gynecol 1975;121:707–13.
6. Westrom LV. Sexually transmitted diseases and infertility. Sex Transm Dis 1994; 21:S32–7.
7. Westrom L, Joesoef R, Reynolds G, et al. Pelvic inflammatory disease and fertility. A cohort study of 1,844 women with laparoscopically verified disease and 657 control women with normal laparoscopic results. Sex Transm Dis 1992;19: 185–92.
8. Houston DE. Evidence for the risk of pelvic endometriosis by age, race and socioeconomic status. Epidemiol Rev 1984;6:167–91.
9. Sensky TE, Liu DT. Endometriosis: associations with menorrhagia, infertility and oral contraceptives. Int J Gynaecol Obstet 1980;17:573–6.
10. Patil M. Assessing tubal damage. J Hum Reprod Sci 2009;2:2–11.
11. Tubercuolsis Fact Sheet No. 104. World Health Organization. 2012.

12. Sutherland AM. The changing pattern of tuberculosis of the female genital tract. A thirty year survey. Arch Gynecol 1983;234:95–101.

13. Sutherland AM. Surgical treatment of tuberculosis of the female genital tract. Br J Obstet Gynaecol 1980;87:610–2.

14. Mueller BA, Daling JR, Moore DE, et al. Appendectomy and the risk of tubal infertility. N Engl J Med 1986;315:1506–8.

15. Mayberry JF, Weterman IT. European survey of fertility and pregnancy in women with Crohn's disease: a case control study by European collaborative group. Gut 1986;27:821–5.

16. Hudson M, Flett G, Sinclair TS, et al. Fertility and pregnancy in inflammatory bowel disease. Int J Gynaecol Obstet 1997;58:229–37.

17. Willoughby CP, Truelove SC. Ulcerative colitis and pregnancy. Gut 1980;21: 469–74.

18. Johnson P, Richard C, Ravid A, et al. Female infertility after ileal pouch-anal anastomosis for ulcerative colitis. Dis Colon Rectum 2004;47:1119–26.

19. Mol BW, Collins JA, Burrows EA, et al. Comparison of hysterosalpingography and laparoscopy in predicting fertility outcome. Hum Reprod 1999;14:1237–42.

20. Moller BR, Allen J, Toft B, et al. Pelvic inflammatory disease after hysterosalpingography associated with *Chlamydia trachomatis* and *Mycoplasma hominis*. Br J Obstet Gynaecol 1984;91:1181–7.

21. Pittaway DE, Winfield AC, Maxson W, et al. Prevention of acute pelvic inflammatory disease after hysterosalpingography: efficacy of doxycycline prophylaxis. Am J Obstet Gynecol 1983;147:623–6.

22. Antibiotic prophylaxis for gynecologic procedures. ACOG Practice Bulletin No. 104. Obstet Gynecol 2009;113:1180–9.

23. Swart P, Mol BW, van der Veen F, et al. The accuracy of hysterosalpingography in the diagnosis of tubal pathology: a meta-analysis. Fertil Steril 1995;64:486–91.

24. Mol BW, Swart P, Bossuyt PM, et al. Reproducibility of the interpretation of hysterosalpingography in the diagnosis of tubal pathology. Hum Reprod 1996;11: 1204–8.

25. Glatstein IZ, Sleeper LA, Lavy Y, et al. Observer variability in the diagnosis and management of the hysterosalpingogram. Fertil Steril 1997;67:233–7.

26. Luttjeboer F, Harada T, Hughes E, et al. Tubal flushing for subfertility. Cochrane Database Syst Rev 2007;(3):CD003718.

27. Watson A, Vandekerckhove P, Lilford R, et al. A meta-analysis of the therapeutic role of oil soluble contrast media at hysterosalpingography: a surprising result? Fertil Steril 1994;61:470–7.

28. Ayida G, Kennedy S, Barlow D, et al. A comparison of patient tolerance of hysterosalpingo-contrast sonography (HyCoSy) with Echovist-200 and X-ray hysterosalpingography for outpatient investigation of infertile women. Ultrasound Obstet Gynecol 1996;7:201–4.

29. Savelli L, Pollastri P, Guerrini M, et al. Tolerability, side effects, and complications of hysterosalpingocontrast sonography (HyCoSy). Fertil Steril 2009;92: 1481–6.

30. Dessole S, Farina M, Rubattu G, et al. Side effects and complications of sonohysterosalpingography. Fertil Steril 2003;80:620–4.

31. Holz K, Becker R, Schurmann R. Ultrasound in the investigation of tubal patency. A meta-analysis of three comparative studies of Echovist-200 including 1007 women. Zentralbl Gynakol 1997;119:366–73.

32. Mardh PA. Tubal factor infertility, with special regard to chlamydial salpingitis. Current Opinion in Infectious Diseases 2004;17:49–52.

33. Mol BW, Dijkman B, Wertheim P, et al. The accuracy of serum chlamydial antibodies in the diagnosis of tubal pathology: a meta-analysis. Fertil Steril 1997; 67:1031–7.
34. Honore GM, Holden AE, Schenken RS. Pathophysiology and management of proximal tubal blockage. Fertil Steril 1999;71:785–95.
35. Thurmond AS, Machan LS, Maubon AJ, et al. A review of selective salpingography and fallopian tube catheterization. Radiographics 2000;20: 1759–68.
36. Thurmond AS, Brandt KR, Gorrill MJ. Tubal obstruction after ligation reversal surgery: results of catheter recanalization. Radiology 1999;210:747–50.
37. Confino E, Friberg J, Gleicher N. Preliminary experience with transcervical balloon tuboplasty. Am J Obstet Gynecol 1988;159:370–5.
38. Maubon A, Rouanet JP, Cover S, et al. Fallopian tube recanalization by selective salpingography: an alternative to more invasive techniques? Hum Reprod 1992; 7:1425–8.
39. Thurmond AS, Rosch J. Nonsurgical fallopian tube recanalization for treatment of infertility. Radiology 1990;174:371–4.
40. Kelekis D, Fezoulidis I, Petsas T, et al. Selective transcervical tubal recanalization under DSA. Rofo 1991;154:354–6 [in German].
41. Thurmond AS. Pregnancies after selective salpingography and tubal recanalization. Radiology 1994;190:11–3.
42. American Fertility Society. The American Fertility Society classification of adnexal adhesions, distal tubal occlusion, tubal occlusion secondary to tubal ligation, tubal pregnancies, Mullerian anomalies and intrauterine adhesions. Fertil Steril 1988;49:944–55.
43. Ahmad G, Watson A, Vandekerckhove P, et al. Techniques for pelvic surgery in subfertility. Cochrane Database Syst Rev 2006;(2):CD000221.
44. Stenchever MADW, Herbst AL, Mishell D. Comprehensive gynecology. 4th edition. St Louis (MO): Mosby; 2001.
45. The role of tubal reconstructive surgery in the era of assisted reproductive technologies. Fertil Steril 2008;90:S250–3.
46. Canis M, Mage G, Pouly JL, et al. Laparoscopic distal tuboplasty: report of 87 cases and a 4-year experience. Fertil Steril 1991;56:616–21.
47. Dlugi AM, Reddy S, Saleh WA, et al. Pregnancy rates after operative endoscopic treatment of total (neosalpingostomy) or near total (salpingostomy) distal tubal occlusion. Fertil Steril 1994;62:913–20.
48. Camus E, Poncelet C, Goffinet F, et al. Pregnancy rates after in-vitro fertilization in cases of tubal infertility with and without hydrosalpinx: a meta-analysis of published comparative studies. Hum Reprod 1999;14:1243–9.
49. Zeyneloglu HB, Arici A, Olive DL. Adverse effects of hydrosalpinx on pregnancy rates after in vitro fertilization-embryo transfer. Fertil Steril 1998;70:492–9.
50. Granot I, Dekel N, Segal I, et al. Is hydrosalpinx fluid cytotoxic? Hum Reprod 1998;13:1620–4.
51. Strandell A, Sjogren A, Bentin-Ley U, et al. Hydrosalpinx fluid does not adversely affect the normal development of human embryos and implantation in vitro. Hum Reprod 1998;13:2921–5.
52. Lessey BA, Castelbaum AJ, Sawin SW, et al. Integrins as markers of uterine receptivity in women with primary unexplained infertility. Fertil Steril 1995;63: 535–42.
53. Meyer WR, Castelbaum AJ, Somkuti S, et al. Hydrosalpinges adversely affect markers of endometrial receptivity. Hum Reprod 1997;12:1393–8.

54. Mansour RT, Aboulghar MA, Serour GI, et al. Fluid accumulation of the uterine cavity before embryo transfer: a possible hindrance for implantation. J In Vitro Fert Embryo Transf 1991;8:157–9.
55. Sowter MC, Akande VA, Williams JA, et al. Is the outcome of in-vitro fertilization and embryo transfer treatment improved by spontaneous or surgical drainage of a hydrosalpinx? Hum Reprod 1997;12:2147–50.
56. Aboulghar MA, Mansour RT, Serour GI, et al. Transvaginal ultrasonic needle guided aspiration of pelvic inflammatory cystic masses before ovulation induction for in vitro fertilization. Fertil Steril 1990;53:311–4.
57. Van Voorhis BJ, Sparks AE, Syrop CH, et al. Ultrasound-guided aspiration of hydrosalpinges is associated with improved pregnancy and implantation rates after in-vitro fertilization cycles. Hum Reprod 1998;13:736–9.
58. Hammadieh N, Coomarasamy A, Ola B, et al. Ultrasound-guided hydrosalpinx aspiration during oocyte collection improves pregnancy outcome in IVF: a randomized controlled trial. Hum Reprod 2008;23:1113–7.
59. Committee opinion: role of tubal surgery in the era of assisted reproductive technology. Fertil Steril 2012;97:539–45.
60. Strandell A, Lindhard A, Waldenstrom U, et al. Hydrosalpinx and IVF outcome: a prospective, randomized multicentre trial in Scandinavia on salpingectomy prior to IVF. Hum Reprod 1999;14:2762–9.
61. Dechaud H, Daures JP, Arnal F, et al. Does previous salpingectomy improve implantation and pregnancy rates in patients with severe tubal factor infertility who are undergoing in vitro fertilization? A pilot prospective randomized study. Fertil Steril 1998;69:1020–5.
62. Kontoravdis A, Makrakis E, Pantos K, et al. Proximal tubal occlusion and salpingectomy result in similar improvement in in vitro fertilization outcome in patients with hydrosalpinx. Fertil Steril 2006;86:1642–9.
63. Johnson N, van Voorst S, Sowter MC, et al. Surgical treatment for tubal disease in women due to undergo in vitro fertilisation. Cochrane Database Syst Rev 2010;(1):CD002125.
64. Moshin V, HA. Reproductive outcome of the proximal tubal occlusion prior to IVF in patients with hydrosalpinx. Hum Reprod 2006;21:i193–4.
65. Stephen EH, CA. Use of infertility services in the United States: 1995. Fam Plann Perspect 2000;32:132–7.
66. Koh CH, Janik GM. Laparoscopic microsurgical tubal anastomosis. Obstet Gynecol Clin North Am 1999;26:189–200, viii.
67. Caillet M, Vandromme J, Rozenberg S, et al. Robotically assisted laparoscopic microsurgical tubal reanastomosis: a retrospective study. Fertil Steril 2010;94:1844–7.
68. Rodgers AK, Goldberg JM, Hammel JP, et al. Tubal anastomosis by robotic compared with outpatient minilaparotomy. Obstet Gynecol 2007;109:1375–80.
69. te Velde ER, Boer ME, Looman CW, et al. Factors influencing success or failure after reversal of sterilization: a multivariate approach. Fertil Steril 1990;54:270–7.
70. Dubuisson JB, Chapron C, Nos C, et al. Sterilization reversal: fertility results. Hum Reprod 1995;10:1145–51.
71. Rock JA, Chang YS, Limpaphayom K, et al. Microsurgical tubal anastomosis: a controlled trial in four Asian centers. Microsurgery 1984;5:95–7.
72. Yoon TK, Sung HR, Kang HG, et al. Laparoscopic tubal anastomosis: fertility outcome in 202 cases. Fertil Steril 1999;72:1121–6.
73. Monteith CW, Berger GS. Normal pregnancy after outpatient tubouterine implantation in patient with Adiana sterilization. Fertil Steril 2011;96:e45–6.

74. Monteith CW, Berger GS. Successful pregnancies after removal of intratubal microinserts. Obstet Gynecol 2012;119:470–2.
75. Gargiulo AR, Nezhat C. Robot-assisted laparoscopy, natural orifice transluminal endoscopy, and single-site laparoscopy in reproductive surgery. Semin Reprod Med 2011;29:155–68.
76. Nezhat C, Saberi NS, Shahmohamady B, et al. Robotic-assisted laparoscopy in gynecological surgery. JSLS 2006;10:317–20.
77. Liu C, Perisic D, Samadi D, et al. Robotic-assisted laparoscopic partial bladder resection for the treatment of infiltrating endometriosis. J Minim Invasive Gynecol 2008;15:745–8.
78. Nezhat C, Morozov V. Robot-assisted laparoscopic presacral neurectomy: feasibility, techniques, and operative outcomes. J Minim Invasive Gynecol 2010;17: 508–12.
79. Barakat EE, Bedaiwy MA, Zimberg S, et al. Robotic-assisted, laparoscopic, and abdominal myomectomy: a comparison of surgical outcomes. Obstet Gynecol 2011;117:256–65.
80. Nezhat C, Lewis M, Kotikela S, et al. Robotic versus standard laparoscopy for the treatment of endometriosis. Fertil Steril 2010;94:2758–60.
81. Nezhat C, Nezhat FR, Nezhat C. Nezhat's operative gynecologic laparoscopy and hysteroscopy. 3rd edition. Cambridge (United Kingdom): Cambridge University Press; 2008.
82. Dharia Patel SP, Steinkampf MP, Whitten SJ, et al. Robotic tubal anastomosis: surgical technique and cost effectiveness. Fertil Steril 2008;90:1175–9.
83. Falcone T, Goldberg JM, Margossian H, et al. Robotic-assisted laparoscopic microsurgical tubal anastomosis: a human pilot study. Fertil Steril 2000;73: 1040–2.
84. Centers for Disease Control and Prevention. 2009 assisted reproductive technology success rates. National Summary and Fertility Clinic Reports. Atlanta (GA): Centers for Disease Control and Prevention; 2011.
85. Karande VC, Korn A, Morris R, et al. Prospective randomized trial comparing the outcome and cost of in vitro fertilization with that of a traditional treatment algorithm as first-line therapy for couples with infertility. Fertil Steril 1999;71:468–75.
86. Pandian Z, Akande VA, Harrild K, et al. Surgery for tubal infertility. Cochrane Database Syst Rev 2008;(3):CD006415.
87. McDonald S, Murphy K, Beyene J, et al. Perinatal outcomes of in vitro fertilization twins: a systematic review and meta-analyses. Am J Obstet Gynecol 2005;193: 141–52.
88. Jackson RA, Gibson KA, Wu YW, et al. Perinatal outcomes in singletons following in vitro fertilization: a meta-analysis. Obstet Gynecol 2004;103:551–63.

A New Approach to Primary Ovarian Insufficiency

Saima Rafique, MBBS, DGO[a], Evelina W. Sterling, PhD[a,b],
Lawrence M. Nelson, MD[c],*

KEYWORDS

- Primary ovarian insufficiency • Premature ovarian failure • Premature menopause
- Infertility • Integrated care

KEY POINTS

- Most women with primary ovarian insufficiency come to clinical attention with oligo/amenorrhea. Take this sign seriously, evaluate it properly, and avoid delay in diagnosis.
- The proper laboratory evaluation of amenorrhea includes a pregnancy test, and if negative, measurement of serum FSH, prolactin, and thyrotropin.
- Women younger than 40 who have 4 months of oligo/amenorrhea and two menopausal serum FSH levels, 1 month apart, meet criteria for primary ovarian insufficiency.
- The indicated tests to determine the mechanism of the disorder include:
  - Karyotype analysis that counts 30 cells so as to uncover mosaic chromosomal abnormalities.
  - Testing for the *FMR1* premutation.
  - Measurement of adrenal antibodies by indirect immunofluorescence and 21- hydroxylase immunoprecipitation tests.
- Primary ovarian insufficiency is a life-altering diagnosis that is highly emotionally charged. Inform women in the office; be supportive and sensitive to their emotions.
- Primary ovarian insufficiency is more than infertility. Physical and emotional health need to be addressed before moving on to plans for creating a family.

Funding Sources: Dr Rafique and Dr Nelson, National Institutes of Health. Dr Sterling, Rachel's Well.
Conflict of Interest: Nil.
[a] Intramural Research Program on Reproductive and Adult Endocrinology, *Eunice Kennedy Shriver* National Institute of Child Health and Human Development, National Institutes of Health, 10 Center Drive, Building 10, CRC, Room 1-3140, Bethesda, MD 20892–1109, USA; [b] Rachel's Well, Project Vital Sign, 1306 Baker Crest Court, McLean, VA 22101, USA; [c] United States Public Health Service, Intramural Research Program on Reproductive and Adult Endocrinology, *Eunice Kennedy Shriver* National Institute of Child Health and Human Development, National Institutes of Health, 10 Center Drive, Building 10, CRC, Room 1-3140, Bethesda, MD 20892-1109, USA
* Corresponding author.
E-mail address: Lawrence_Nelson@nih.gov

Obstet Gynecol Clin N Am 39 (2012) 567–586
http://dx.doi.org/10.1016/j.ogc.2012.09.007
0889-8545/12/$ – see front matter Published by Elsevier Inc.

INTRODUCTION

Recently the National Institutes of Health convened a stakeholders meeting on primary ovarian insufficiency to explore ways in which to advance the field. The published report stressed the need for an integrative approach.[1] Women with primary ovarian insufficiency face the acute shock of the diagnosis; associated stigma of infertility; grief from the death of dreams; anxiety and depression from the disruption of life plans; confusion around the cause; symptoms of estrogen deficiency; worry over the associated potential medical sequelae, such as reduced bone density and cardiovascular risk; and the uncertain future that all of these factors create.[2,3] Evidence supports a role for a collaborative care model as a method to improve medical outcomes, reduce costs, and to do so in a way that clinicians find satisfying.[4–6] This approach should be combined with the development of a public health knowledge network on primary ovarian insufficiency.[7,8] This knowledge network would form the central component of a community of practice for the condition.[9,10]

The authors' research team now includes a reproductive endocrinologist, reproductive psychiatrist, medical endocrinologist, occupational therapist, recreational therapist, nutritionist, chaplain, and social worker. They have learned that they need to know the patient at a personal level to care for them appropriately. Before evaluation, all of their patients answer a series of questions in writing about themselves and how primary ovarian insufficiency has affected their lives (**Box 1**). The authors call this "The Patient Narrative" and share it in confidence with the entire team. This practice has changed their team dynamics and given greater meaning to their work.

For most women the infertility associated with the diagnosis is the most upsetting component of the disorder (**Box 2**).[11] However, primary ovarian insufficiency involves many aspects of a woman's life. It is a serious chronic disease that requires long-term management. Chronic illnesses change people's lives. Patients and their caregivers are abruptly confronted with a restricted and uncertain future. They also acquire

---

Box 1
Patient narrative questions for women with primary ovarian insufficiency to answer in writing

a. What would you like us to know about you as a person?

b. How would you like your life to change in the next six months?

c. What are your aspirations for your life in the long term?

d. What gives your life meaning and purpose?

e. If nothing changed in your life right now what would that mean to you?

f. What were your dreams about your future family life before you found out that you have primary ovarian insufficiency?

g. How has primary ovarian insufficiency affected your life?

h. Please give us an example of a difficult situation in your life from the past (other than your diagnosis of primary ovarian insufficiency) and explain to us how you coped with that.

i. How do you cope with the diagnosis of primary ovarian insufficiency?

j. What fears do you have about the diagnosis of primary ovarian insufficiency and how it will affect your future?

k. What fears do you have about your visit here?

l. Is there anything else that you want us to know about you?

Box 2
Worries articulated by a patient advocate with primary ovarian insufficiency

- What if my pregnancy test never turns positive?
- What if I never fill my baby scrapbook page?
- What if my infertility robs me of my sexiness and I'm never "in the mood again"?
- What if we finally save enough money for our one egg donation cycle and it fails?
- What if we can't afford to adopt?
- What if I can't counter the thought that I had to "buy" a baby?
- What if I have to read another pregnancy announcement in an online social media today?
- What if we have to learn to live child free… with a smile?
- What if he leaves me for a fertile woman?
- What if I never let go of the resentment and jealousy of the woman who got to do this naturally?
- What if I lose myself along the way?
- What if I stop defining myself by my infertility?
- What if I stop hiding behind my fears?
- What if I stop hiding behind my grief?
- What if I redefine what it means to be a woman?
- What if I redefine what it means to be a mother?
- What if I redefine what it means to be a family?
- What if I let go of the doubt, the fear, the worry, and the self-judgment for one day?
- What if I lived in the moment rather than in an uncertain future?

Courtesy of Keiko Zoll, writer and founder of TheInfertilityVoice.com; with permission.

---

new burdens associated with managing the disease.[6,12] In most cases couples discover they are infertile in a gradual manner after many failed attempts at conception. In stark contrast, for most women with primary ovarian insufficiency knowledge of the diagnosis arrives abruptly and unexpectedly as part of an evaluation for oligo/amenorrhea or polymenorrhea, in many cases even before they have a partner or have even attempted conception.[13]

"Devastated," "shocked," and "confused" are the most common words women use to describe their feelings in the hours after being informed of this diagnosis.[14] These are words that describe emotional trauma. Many clinicians resolve during their early years of training to learn from their patients, listen attentively to them, and to provide culturally appropriate, patient-centered care. Then the tyranny of reality takes over.[15] The past few decades have brought incredible progress to the scientific underpinnings of reproductive medicine. Some of these technologies have taken precedence over a critical skill of the compassionate clinician: the art of listening to the patient.[16] A recent report that compared physician career satisfaction with their chosen specialty showed that obstetrics and gynecology scored unfavorably.[17] Similarly, most women with primary ovarian insufficiency get their diagnosis from a gynecologist, and most of them are unsatisfied with how they were informed about it.[14] A focus on problem-solving often blinds physicians to emotional issues in their patients and themselves.[18]

It seems that both sides of the equation in this dilemma see room for improvement in the shared experience of primary ovarian insufficiency.[19]

OVARIAN PHYSIOLOGY

Estradiol is by far the most potent of the three major natural human estrogens: estradiol, estrone, and estriol. The dominant graafian follicle, which develops anew each month within the ovary, is the main source of estradiol in reproductive-aged women. The graafian follicle develops from microscopic primordial follicles, the structures in the ovary where oocytes are stored. The primordial follicle number peaks at 6 to 7 million by 20 weeks of gestation in a human female fetus.[20] Thereafter they rapidly undergo atresia leaving only 1 to 2 million oocytes at birth. At puberty there are only 300,000 of the original 6 to 7 million left, of these only 400 to 500 oocytes are released during ovulation in the entire reproductive life.[21] Menopause, the permanent cessation of menses, occurs because of depletion of functional primordial follicles. The mean age of menopause is 50 ± 4 years and if it occurs before 40 years it is considered premature.[22]

THE CLINICAL PROBLEM

Primary ovarian insufficiency is the preferred term for this condition.[2,23,24] The term was initially used in 1942 by Fuller Albright, who first described the condition and who many consider to be the father of modern endocrinology. His research report made it clear that the amenorrhea was caused by impaired ovarian function as the primary cause rather than a pituitary disorder (secondary cause).[23,25] Other terms, such as premature ovarian failure, premature menopause, early menopause, hypergonadotropic hypogonadism, ovarian dysgenesis, and hypergonadotropic amenorrhea, have also been used in the literature to describe the condition.[1]

Presentation

Primary ovarian insufficiency affects 1 in 10,000 women by age 20, 1 in 1000 by age 30, and 1 in 100 by age 40.[26] Although primary amenorrhea may be the initial symptom in 10% of cases, more often patients present with irregular menstrual cycles in the form of oligo/amenorrhea, polymenorrhea, or dysfunctional uterine bleeding after having attained normal puberty and having established regular menstrual cycles.[27]

Diagnostic Criteria

To meet diagnostic criteria for primary ovarian insufficiency patients need to be younger than 40 years of age, have experienced 4 months of oligo/amenorrhea, and on investigation be found to have two serum follicle-stimulating hormone (FSH) levels in the menopausal range, obtained at least a month apart (**Box 3**).[27–29] Evidence has

---

Box 3
Criteria to establish the diagnosis of primary ovarian insufficiency

Younger than 40 years of age

Oligo/amenorrhea lasting 4 months

Two FSH levels in the menopausal range, obtained at least a month apart

Data from Nelson LM. Clinical practice. Primary ovarian insufficiency. N Engl J Med 2009;360(6):606–14.

demonstrated that most women with primary ovarian insufficiency experience intermittent ovarian function rather than complete cessation of ovarian function. Therefore, most of these patients are expected to have irregular and unpredictable menses rather than complete amenorrhea. Hence, a period of complete amenorrhea is not required to make the diagnosis.[2]

Mechanisms

Primary ovarian insufficiency can be caused by follicular dysfunction or follicular depletion.[28] Although in follicular depletion there are no follicles left in the ovary, in follicular dysfunction even though there are follicles in the ovary they are unable to function normally. The cause of dysfunction may be a signal defect in FSH or luteinizing hormone receptor function[30] or G protein mutation,[31] enzyme deficiency,[32] ovarian autoimmunity,[33] or the development of luteinized graafian follicles related to low follicle cohort size.[34] Follicle depletion can be caused by insufficient initial follicular count, spontaneous accelerated follicular loss as in Turner syndrome,[35] or environmental toxin–induced follicular loss.[36]

Primary ovarian insufficiency can be nonsyndromic or it may be a part of a syndrome. Nonsyndromic primary ovarian insufficiency has been associated with several genes, such as bone morphogenic protein 15,[37] diaphanous homolog 2,[38] and inhibin alpha subunit.[39] It may also occur because of structural abnormalities in the X chromosome.[40] In 90% of cases the cause remains enigmatic.[2]

Evaluation

To start, take a detailed menstrual history, ask about symptoms of estrogen deficiency, and enquire about symptoms related to potentially associated diseases (**Box 4**). Most commonly, aberrant menstruation is the presenting complaint, although symptoms of estrogen deficiency, such as vasomotor symptoms, mood disturbances, change in sleep cycle, and dyspareunia caused by atrophic vaginitis, may be present. Primary ovarian insufficiency may also be a part of an autoimmune polyglandular syndrome; patients should be questioned and educated on symptoms of hypothyroidism and adrenal insufficiency. It may also be associated with dry eye syndrome,[41] myasthenia gravis, rheumatoid arthritis, and systemic lupus erythematosus.[33] Although most cases occur sporadically, in approximately 10% to 15% of cases there is an affected first-degree relative, so a well-structured family history is important.[42] A history of intellectual disability, dementia, tremor, or ataxia in the family may point to premutation in *FMR1* gene, responsible for fragile X syndrome, the most common

---

Box 4
Tests indicated in the evaluation of confirmed primary ovarian insufficiency

Karyotype (count 30 cells)

Adrenal antibodies

　　21-hydroxylase (CYP21) by immunoprecipitation

　　Indirect immunofluorescence

FMR1 premutation

Pelvic ultrasound

Bone mineral density

Data from Nelson LM. Clinical practice. Primary ovarian insufficiency. N Engl J Med 2009;360(6):606–14.

form of heritable intellectual disability.[43] Physical examination may reveal the stigmata of associated disorders, such as autoimmune polyglandular syndrome type 1, thyroid disease, adrenal insufficiency, or Turner syndrome.

Most patients present with secondary amenorrhea. The evaluation of amenorrhea begins with a pregnancy test. After pregnancy is ruled out a complete history should determine if the amenorrhea could be the earliest manifestation of a decline in general health, such as uncontrolled diabetes mellitus, an underlying condition, such as celiac disease, excessive exercise, inadequate caloric intake, emotional stress, or prior radiation therapy or chemotherapy. Is there galactorrhea or signs of androgen excess? It is inappropriate to attribute amenorrhea to stress without further evaluation. Indicated laboratory tests in the evaluation of secondary amenorrhea include serum prolactin, FSH, and thyrotropin levels.[44]

A menopausal range FSH should be repeated in 1 month to confirm the diagnosis of primary ovarian insufficiency. After the diagnosis is confirmed the findings should be discussed with the patient at a return office visit rather than by telephone. This information is highly emotionally charged. The indicated tests to determine the mechanism of the disorder after the diagnosis of primary ovarian insufficiency is established include (1) karyotype analysis that counts 30 cells so as to uncover mosaic chromosomal abnormalities, (2) offer testing for the FMR1 premutation, and (3) measurement of adrenal antibodies by indirect immunofluorescence and 21-hydroxylase immunoprecipitation tests.

The fragile X premutation is found in approximately 2% of women who have isolated spontaneous 46, XX primary ovarian insufficiency and in 14% of women with a familial presentation; the premutation increases the risk of conceiving a child with intellectual disability because of fragile X syndrome.[43] Approximately 4% of women with primary ovarian insufficiency screen positive for adrenal antibodies, which indicates that steroidogenic cell autoimmunity and lymphocytic autoimmune oophoritis are the mechanism of the disorder.[45] Ovarian antibody tests lack proved specificity and are not indicated.[46] Ovarian biopsy is not indicated in the evaluation of this condition. Because of sampling error pregnancy is known to occur even after reports of no follicles present on biopsy.[47] A pelvic ultrasound is also indicated to detect those women with primary ovarian insufficiency who have enlarged multicystic ovaries, as can be seen in 17,20-desmolase deficiency and autoimmune oophoritis.[45]

MANAGEMENT
Overview

Infertility is best defined from an emotional perspective as a socially constructed life crisis.[48] Viewed from this perspective it is not primarily a medical disorder but a disruption in life plans. Evidence has demonstrated that women who have been evaluated for infertility and fail to conceive a child are twice as likely to commit suicide as women who subsequently had a child.[49] The authors' team has lived through the experience of having one of their patients with autoimmune primary ovarian insufficiency commit suicide. In the ensuing court proceedings her diary made it clear that the infertility associated with her condition was a major factor in the tragedy.[50]

Primary ovarian insufficiency is a chronic disorder that not only disrupts the dreams a woman has around her fertility but the shock of the diagnosis and the stigma attached with it may leave her alone, suffering silently in grief.[51] Associated medical conditions may also surface as a part of the evaluation. Women with primary ovarian insufficiency are also susceptible to future health risks of decreased bone mineral density and increased cardiovascular morbidity related to estrogen deficiency.[52]

Primary ovarian insufficiency is most commonly diagnosed as part of evaluation for other gynecologic complains, such as irregular menses, so the diagnosis usually comes as a surprise and leaves many women with the condition feeling helpless, hopeless, and frustrated with their medical care.[53] Frequently the diagnosis comes after seeing more than three clinicians who did not take the menstrual irregularity seriously enough to evaluate the situation by measuring FSH.[13] Furthermore, most women are dissatisfied with the care they receive for primary ovarian insufficiency even after the diagnosis is made.[14] Most women with the diagnosis feel unprepared for the shock and want their clinician to spend more time with them to give them more information, medical guidance, and emotional support.[14] These women experience emotional distress, anxiety, and depression and are longing for emotional support and professional guidance to help them find their new path forward.[54] It is crucial that clinicians provide integrative care that covers the different aspects of their health that are at risk related to the diagnosis.

Emotional Health

The diagnosis of primary ovarian insufficiency and the associated unanticipated infertility seriously disrupts life plans.[53] Evidence suggests that people with infertility suffer from a higher degree of psychological stress.[48,55] Studies specifically conducted on women with primary ovarian insufficiency demonstrate lower self-esteem and increased shyness and social anxiety.[56] For many women, the grief response is equivalent to the loss of a loved one.[57] Such unexpected losses are frequently associated with increased psychological morbidity and higher rates of depression.[58–64] Schmidt and colleagues[65] in their study showed that women with primary ovarian insufficiency had a higher frequency of depression and greater lifetime risk of depression. Thus, these women should be evaluated for underlying depression and offered expert care, should it be present. Women with primary ovarian insufficiency also have a lower perceived social support and may be isolating themselves.[66] It is important for clinicians to educate these patients and guide them to the resources that could help them in their emotional healing. If appropriate and with patient's consent, informing partners and other family members regarding the challenges these women face can help patients create an environment of trust, warmth, and support at home. When needed, community-based resources, such as couples counseling and professionally guided social services, might help in their emotional healing. The authors have found that when making the diagnosis of primary ovarian insufficiency in adolescents, taking a family systems approach is beneficial.[67]

Meaning and Purpose

Maslow's hierarchy of needs is a theory that focuses on describing the stages of human growth from a developmental psychology perspective.[68] Wellness includes the psychological health that permits thriving despite the existential difficulties and challenges in life. Wellness includes such things as pursuing meaningful goals, growing and developing as a person, and establishing quality ties to others.[69] There exists what has been termed the "parental paradox." This paradox has been used as an example to describe the difference between happiness and meaning. First, in retrospect parents usually report that they are very glad they had children, but parents living with children usually score very low on happiness indicators. Raising children may decrease parental happiness but increase parental meaning in life.[70] Viktor Frankl changed Maslow's paradigm. He placed "self-transcendence" at the top of a newly ordered Maslow's hierarchy. Maslow placed "self-actualization" at the top. Frankl[71] argued in his book *From Death Camp to Existentialism* that self-actualization is not possible as long as the self is the center of action. According to Frankl, one must move beyond self interest to reach the top of the human development pyramid.

For most women having children is a major life goal, and having this goal disrupted by the diagnosis of primary ovarian insufficiency is difficult and challenging. Research has shown that women with primary ovarian insufficiency who score higher on a measure of meaning and purpose have fewer symptoms of anxiety and depression, higher positive affect, and lower negative affect.[51] Meaning and purpose in life is a motivational force during adversity. In a recent study women with primary ovarian insufficiency scored adversely compared with control women on all tested measures of affect. Women who had greater goal flexibility and a stronger sense of meaning and purpose in life experienced greater positive effect.[51] Helping these women find new avenues to meaning and purpose may help them cope better. For many women with primary ovarian insufficiency providing spiritual care can be a path to new meaning and purpose, and likely fewer symptoms of anxiety and depression.[72] Ventura and colleagues[73] provide evidence that women with primary ovarian insufficiency who scored better on a measure of spiritual well-being also scored better on a measure of functional well-being. Rearranging goals and finding strength in spiritual care can infuse patients with positive energy to move ahead and persevere.

Hormone Replacement

Most women with primary ovarian insufficiency need hormone replacement to reduce symptoms of estrogen deficiency, such as vaginal dryness and vasomotor instability. In contrast to normally menopausal women in their 50s, the need for hormone replacement in these young women clearly extends beyond the need for symptom relief. There is undoubtedly a role for continued hormone replacement until age 50 years in these young women (50 is the average age of menopause). Evidence suggests this is justified to protect them from development of serious morbidity and earlier mortality related to prolonged estrogen deficiency. Early menopause has been associated with an increased incidence of fractures and increased total mortality and mortality caused by ischemic heart disease.[74–77] It is invalid to apply the results of the Women's Health Initiative to young women with primary ovarian insufficiency in determining the risk/benefit ratio for women of reproductive age. The Women's Health Initiative demonstrated that combined hormone therapy (estrogen with progestin) increased the risk of cardiovascular events in menopausal women, but importantly, the participants in this study were, on average, 63 years of age.[78] The age difference between the women in the Women's Health Initiative study and young women with primary ovarian insufficiency is of paramount import. The Women's Health Initiative was not a primary prevention study of cardiovascular disease. Such a study should have begun at the time women began developing estrogen deficiency. For many women this transition to an estrogen-deficient state could have begun 10 to 20 years before age 63. Primary ovarian insufficiency in young women is a pathologic condition in which women have lower serum estradiol levels compared with their peers of similar age; in contrast, menopause is a physiologic condition of older women.[2] It is important for the clinician to keep this in mind when discussing the risk/benefit ratio of hormone therapy in young women with primary ovarian insufficiency.[2,23]

The main goal of hormone therapy for women with primary ovarian insufficiency is to mimic normal ovarian function with regard to estradiol replacement. The average serum estradiol level during the menstrual cycle in normal women is approximately 100 pg/mm.[79] Transdermal and transvaginal replacement of 100 µg/day of estradiol achieves physiologic blood levels in this range and provides adequate symptomatic relief. Transdermal or transvaginal route of administration has a lower risk of vascular thromboembolism compared with oral estrogen.[80–82] Evidence supports the addition of cyclical medroxyprogesterone acetate at the dose of 10 mg/day for 12 days each month because this guards against the potential risk of endometrial cancer by inducing full secretory endometrium and sloughing on a regular basis.[83,84] A menstrual calendar should be maintained and a pregnancy test should be done if menses are delayed, because conception can occur in 5% to 10% of these women. Most women with primary ovarian insufficiency are experiencing ongoing intermittent ovarian function.[2,85] If pregnancy occurs the estradiol-progestin replacement should be discontinued. Oral contraceptives are not recommended as first-line hormone replacement in women with primary ovarian insufficiency; they provide more steroid hormone than is needed for physiologic replacement and are associated with an increased risk of thromboembolic events related to the first pass effect on the liver.[2] A major advantage of transdermal and transvaginal estradiol replacement is the avoidance of this first pass effect on the liver.

Professional Society Recommendations

The American Society for Reproductive Medicine and the International Menopause Society have recommended estrogen-replacement therapy for women with primary ovarian insufficiency.[44,86] There are also recommendations from several professional organizations advising that patients with primary ovarian insufficiency be offered testing for a premutation in the FMR1 gene.[87–89]

Bone Health

Compared with control women, women with primary ovarian insufficiency have reduced bone mineral density.[90] No evidence-based guidelines have been developed specifically for women with primary ovarian insufficiency with regard to maintaining bone health, but it is reasonable to follow the guidelines put forth by the North American Menopause Society.[91] Hypogonadism is a risk factor for osteoporosis, so patients with primary ovarian insufficiency need to be informed about this and monitored regarding their compliance with how to reduce this risk. They should be encouraged to practice a variety of weight-bearing exercises, such as walking, jogging, stair climbing, and resistance training.[92] Intake of 1200 mg of elemental calcium per day is recommended.[91] It has been recommended that adults with inadequate sun exposure take at least 800 to 1000 IU of vitamin D per day.[93] Adequate vitamin D status is defined as a serum 25-hyroxyvitamin D level of 30 ng/mm or higher.[93] Because of the uncertain effects of bisphosphonates on fetus and their long skeletal half-life these agents are not recommended in women who might subsequently conceive.[94]

Genetic Health

In 10% to 15% of cases women with this disorder have an affected first-degree relative. A family history of fragile X syndrome, intellectual disability, dementia, tremor and ataxia, or symptoms like those of Parkinson's disease raises the possibility that a fragile X premutation might be the cause of the primary ovarian insufficiency. Patients with a strong family history suggesting this possibility should be offered genetic counseling before the FMR1 test is performed. This gives them a head start in thinking about how to inform the rest of the family in the event they are found to carry the premutation.

Nutrition

An assessment by a nutritionist helps these women chart a balanced diet specific to their choices and requirements. Familiarizing them with foods rich in calcium, educating them about healthy food options to maintain cardiovascular health, and guidance about vitamin D intake are important for long-term health. Women who desire to conceive should be encouraged to get ready for pregnancy by making healthy food decisions. They should be made aware of the detrimental effects of alcohol[95,96] and smoking[97] on the fetus and pregnancy and should be inspired to make necessary changes. Foods rich in folic acid and preconception folic acid supplements to prevent neural tube defects should be offered because pregnancy usually occurs unexpectedly in women with primary ovarian insufficiency.[98] Women with diabetes or underlying celiac disease get additional benefit from nutritional guidance.[99]

Associated Conditions

Adrenal insufficiency, also known as Addison disease, is a potentially fatal disorder. One report uncovered asymptomatic adrenal insufficiency in approximately 3% of women with primary ovarian insufficiency,[100] an increase of at least a 100-fold risk compared with the general population. Testing for the presence of adrenal autoimmunity by measuring adrenal antibodies is recommended in all women with primary ovarian insufficiency.[100] Patients who test positive for adrenal autoimmunity should have an annual corticotropin stimulation test to assess adrenal function. All women with primary ovarian insufficiency should be informed about the symptoms of adrenal insufficiency and instructed to seek out evaluation should such symptoms develop.

Thyroid autoimmunity, mainly Hashimoto thyroiditis, is also more common in women with primary ovarian insufficiency; prevalence rates of 14% to 27% have been reported.[33,101] Compared with control women, women with primary ovarian insufficiency also have an increased incidence of dry-eye syndrome, seen in about 20% of these patients.[41] Referral to an ophthalmologist can be quite beneficial. Although primary ovarian insufficiency has also been associated with other autoimmune diseases, such as myasthenia gravis, rheumatoid arthritis, and systemic lupus erythematosus, because of the limited frequency of associations testing for these and other autoimmune disorders should be based only on indication by the presence of relevant symptoms and signs.

FAMILY PLANNING

Childbearing and motherhood are celebrated by most societies and couples who electively or otherwise decide not to raise children carry a burden of stigma (**Box 5**).[102-104] Even the most developed and modern societies are touched by pronatalism and pressure for reproductive conformity.[105] Couples facing infertility, in addition to

---

Box 5
Family planning options in primary ovarian insufficiency

- Await spontaneous conception
- Child-free living
- Adoption
- Foster children
- Oocyte donation
- Embryo donation

Data from Baker V. Life plans and family-building options for women with primary ovarian insufficiency. Semin Reprod Med 2011;29(4):362–72.

experiencing stigma, frequently experience a sense of loss of meaning and purpose in life[106] and feelings of loss of control and isolation.[107,108]

Although fertility may be a major concern for many women with primary ovarian insufficiency, it is important to point out that this is not true of all women, and certainly in many cases the diagnosis is made years before creating a family is an issue for the patient. It is important to meet the patient where she is in this regard rather than assuming that parenthood is her current goal. As one of our patients lamented after reading one of our publications,

> As someone who suffers from this condition, I was happy to see mention of the emotional aspects that it involves. But I wish the medical community would stop pushing donor eggs or adoption as solutions to our problems. I understand these work for some people, but they are far from a cure. We feel lost and broken, with very little quality of life.

It is important to make clear to patients that spontaneous remission of primary ovarian insufficiency is not rare, and that unexpected pregnancy occurs in about 5% to 10% of cases.[85] Although uncommon, remissions may in some cases even last for years with return of regular ovulatory menstrual cycles.[28] Presently, there are no validated markers that are predictive of remission and there are no therapies proved safe and effective in restoring ovarian function and fertility in this condition. Women with primary ovarian insufficiency who wish to avoid pregnancy should not rely on the oral contraceptive. The effectiveness of these agents has not been studied in this population. There are reports of women with this condition conceiving while complying with an oral contraceptive regimen.[109] It is possible that contraceptive failures occur in this population because oral contraceptives fail to adequately suppress the characteristically high serum FSH levels seen in these patients.[2]

It is the clinician's responsibility to assess the patient's general health with regard to the effects of primary ovarian insufficiency before helping them down the road to parenthood. For example, moving to egg donation in a woman with unrecognized major depression or asymptomatic adrenal insufficiency obviously would not be in the best interest of the woman or the child to be conceived. The appropriate time for the clinician to raise questions about creating a family, by either traditional or high-technology methods, is after having established that the she is endocrinologically healthy with regard to adrenal and thyroid function and, importantly, adequately recovered emotionally from the news of the diagnosis.[3]

Some couples desire parenthood but are uncomfortable with adoption or reproductive technology as a solution. They are content to define their family as the couple and accept the real, albeit low, chance that they will conceive without medical intervention. Because ovarian function is intermittent and unpredictable, attempts to time intercourse are not indicated. Couples who want to optimize their chances for conception should have intercourse two or three times a week to ensure that sperm are present should an ovulation occur (sperm can survive in the female genital tract for 3 days).[110] Although the hormone-replacement regimen induces regular menstrual cycles this does not mean that ovulation occur on Day 14 of the induced cycle. Ovulations are still intermittent and unpredictable.

For couples ready to pursue parenthood actively the options are adoption, foster parenthood, egg donation, and embryo donation. In the special circumstance in which the patient has an identical twin with normal ovarian function ovarian transplantation is possible.[111] The success of egg donations is primarily dependent on the age of the egg donor, so there is no medical urgency to proceed to egg donation. Rates of pregnancy with this method are similar among older and younger women.[112] There is some evidence to suggest that with egg donation there is a higher incidence of pregnancy complications, such as postpartum hemorrhage, small for gestational age, pregnancy-induced hypertension, and a minimal increase in the rate of birth malformations.[113-115] However, for most couples these risks are not of a great enough magnitude to decide against the approach. Embryo donation has comparable results with egg donation and is less expensive.[116]

PLANS FOR ONGOING MANAGEMENT

Primary ovarian insufficiency is a serious chronic disease that requires ongoing management in an integrated and collaborative manner. The combination of the associated emotional sequelae including loss of meaning and purpose in life around disruption of plans for a family, need for hormone replacement, concerns regarding long-term bone health and cardiovascular health, and the potential for associated hypothyroidism and adrenal insufficiency cut across diverse sets of expertise.[50] A model of care for primary ovarian insufficiency should be developed that combines an integrative and collaborative approach in a way that patients and clinicians find satisfying.[1,4-6]

To provide continuity of care an individual should be identified who will serve as the patient's "personal health advocate." This individual would work with the patient to develop a written ongoing management plan that integrates the diverse aspects of care these women require. The personal health advocate would assist in transition from one phase of care to another and make the necessary arrangements for care.[117,118] For many women the most challenging part of the disorder is making decisions about their plans for creating a family in view of the diagnosis. Greil[48] has pointed out that learning of infertility precipitates a "socially constructed life crisis" that must be navigated. Primary ovarian insufficiency is one of the special circumstances in which women may learn about their infertility even before attempting conception, sometimes even during adolescence.[67] The authors have found that including a social worker on the team adds a unique perspective and brings expertise that can link patient to community resources on wellness, individual and couples counseling, spiritual care, financial management, support groups that are professionally monitored, and generally provide a resource for finding creative solutions to unmet needs.[119,120]

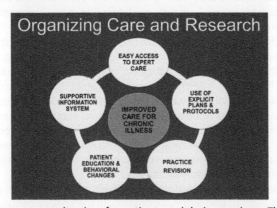

Fig. 1. Chronic illnesses create burdens for patients and their caregivers. They also restrict life and create uncertainty about the future. Successful interventions to reorganize research and care delivery in chronic diseases share common characteristics as illustrated. (*Data from* Wagner EH, Austin BT, Von Korff M. Organizing care for patients with chronic illness. Milbank Q 1996;74(4):511-44.)

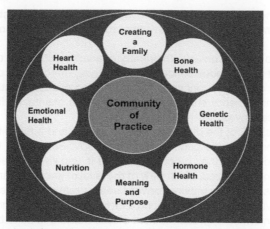

Fig. 2. The large circle defines the domain of the community of primary ovarian insufficiency. This includes all women with primary ovarian insufficiency that at any one time may be focused on entirely different aspects of their chronic disease. The disorder is much more than infertility. The red circle in the center represents the community of practice that serves these women. A community of practice is a group of people who provide services to the larger community. By sharing information and experiences with each other they develop personally and professionally, and can provide better care to the larger community.

EYE TO THE FUTURE

The new paradigm for studying and treating primary ovarian insufficiency is taking a community of practice approach.[10] This concept is little known in the medical community, but communities of practice have been referred to as the organizational structure of the future by the business community.[9] The community of practice provides a construct in which stakeholders can work collaboratively to tackle complex, multidimensional, and hierarchical problems despite limited resources. Such a community of practice for primary ovarian insufficiency came together in an event organized by the National Institutes of Health.[1,10] A major goal of the primary ovarian insufficiency community is to create a knowledge network.[7,8] Knowledge networks disseminate ideas, catalyze creative thinking, and serve as an engine for progress and change that advance research and improve patient care. Rachel's Well, a not-for-profit entity, serves as the umbrella organization for the primary ovarian insufficiency community of practice and associated knowledge network (http://www. rachelswell.org/).[1] The organization promotes an integrative model of care delivery and research that places the patient at the center of all efforts. Rachel's Well advocates a wellness approach to primary ovarian insufficiency. Such an approach creates synergy between the powers of spiritual care and highly technical care and requires major reorganization to a new model of research and care delivery (**Figs. 1** and **2**).[6,12]

SUMMARY

Primary ovarian insufficiency is a life-altering diagnosis and many patients consider the diagnosis to be a threat to their identity as a woman. The diagnosis is much more than infertility. There are effects on emotional health, physical health, and spiritual wellness.

To make the diagnosis of primary ovarian insufficiency in a timely manner one must take oligo/amenorrhea seriously and evaluate it appropriately. Women with primary ovarian insufficiency are deficient in the ovarian hormones and estradiol should be administered by transdermal and transvaginal routes with oral medroxyprogesterone acetate.

It is important to inform women with primary ovarian insufficiency that there is a 5% to 10% chance of spontaneous conception. However, there are no proved strategies for increasing the chance of conception by improving ovarian function. Women with primary ovarian insufficiency should be encouraged to maintain a lifestyle that optimizes bone and cardiovascular health.

The emotional shock of the diagnosis can be severe and it takes time for husband and wife to get on the same page about next steps. Some time to permit natural conception to occur while they process the grief is usually in order. The amount of time needs to be individualized, but in view of the level of grief that can be encountered 3 years of processing before moving forward seems reasonable. Setting a time such as this before moving forward with creating a family takes the pressure off and permits a measured and informed approach to next steps. Some decide to be the completed family together as a couple without children. If no spontaneous conception occurs in the allotted adjustment time interval, adoption, foster children, egg donation, and embryo donation are the options for those who want to be parents.

ACKNOWLEDGMENTS

The authors thank Peter and Cindy Catches of Oceti Wakan (http://www.ocetiwakan.org/) for valuable discussions regarding the spiritual care of women with primary ovarian insufficiency. This work was supported in part by Rachel's Well, Inc (http://www.rachelswell.org/) and the Intramural Research Program of the National Institutes of Health (http://irp.nih.gov/).

REFERENCES

1. Cooper AR, Baker VL, Sterling EW, et al. The time is now for a new approach to primary ovarian insufficiency. Fertil Steril 2011;95(6):1890–7.
2. Nelson LM. Clinical practice. Primary ovarian insufficiency. N Engl J Med 2009; 360(6):606–14.
3. Sterling EW, Nelson LM. From victim to survivor to thriver: helping women with primary ovarian insufficiency integrate recovery, self-management, and wellness. Semin Reprod Med 2011;29(4):353–61.
4. Levine S, Unutzer J, Yip JY, et al. Physicians' satisfaction with a collaborative disease management program for late-life depression in primary care. Gen Hosp Psychiatry 2005;27(6):383–91.
5. Katon WJ, Lin EH, Von Korff M, et al. Collaborative care for patients with depression and chronic illnesses. N Engl J Med 2010;363(27):2611–20.
6. Katon W, Russo J, Lin EH, et al. Cost-effectiveness of a multicondition collaborative care intervention: a randomized controlled trial. Arch Gen Psychiatry 2012;69(5):506–14.
7. Arora S, Geppert CM, Kalishman S, et al. Academic health center management of chronic diseases through knowledge networks: Project ECHO. Acad Med 2007;82(2):154–60.
8. Arora S, Thornton K, Murata G, et al. Outcomes of treatment for hepatitis C virus infection by primary care providers. N Engl J Med 2011;364(23):2199–207.
9. Wenger EC, Snyder WM. Communities of practice: the organizational frontier. Harv Bus Rev 2000;78:139–45.

10. Frankfurter D. A new paradigm for studying and treating primary ovarian insufficiency: the community of practice. Fertil Steril 2011;95(6):1899–900 [discussion: 1902].
11. Zoll K. What IF? A portrait of infertility. Available at: http://vimeo.com/11214833. 2010. Accessed October 16, 2011.
12. Wagner EH, Austin BT, Von Korff M. Organizing care for patients with chronic illness. Milbank Q 1996;74(4):511–44.
13. Alzubaidi NH, Chapin HL, Vanderhoof VH, et al. Meeting the needs of young women with secondary amenorrhea and spontaneous premature ovarian failure. Obstet Gynecol 2002;99(5 Pt 1):720–5.
14. Groff AA, Covington SN, Halverson LR, et al. Assessing the emotional needs of women with spontaneous premature ovarian failure. Fertil Steril 2005;83(6):1734–41.
15. Henry SG. A piece of my mind. The tyranny of reality. JAMA 2011;305(4):338–9.
16. Levinson W, Pizzo PA. Patient-physician communication: it's about time. JAMA 2011;305(17):1802–3.
17. Leigh JP, Tancredi DJ, Kravitz RL. Physician career satisfaction within specialties. BMC Health Serv Res 2009;9:166.
18. Lamberg L. "If I work hard(er), I will be loved." Roots of physician stress explored. JAMA 1999;282(1):13–4.
19. Conigliaro RL. A piece of my mind. Satisfaction? JAMA 2005;293(18):2193.
20. Peters H, Byskov AG, Grinsted J. Follicular growth in fetal and prepubertal ovaries of humans and other primates. Clin Endocrinol Metab 1978;7(3):469–85.
21. Himelstein-Braw R, Byskov AG, Peters H, et al. Follicular atresia in the infant human ovary. J Reprod Fertil 1976;46(1):55–9.
22. van Noord PA, Dubas JS, Dorland M, et al. Age at natural menopause in a population-based screening cohort: the role of menarche, fecundity, and lifestyle factors. Fertil Steril 1997;68(1):95–102.
23. Welt CK. Primary ovarian insufficiency: a more accurate term for premature ovarian failure. Clin Endocrinol (Oxf) 2008;68(4):499–509.
24. De Vos M, Devroey P, Fauser BC. Primary ovarian insufficiency. Lancet 2010; 376(9744):911–21.
25. Albright F, Smith PH, Fraser R. A syndrome characterized by primary ovarian insufficiency and decreased stature. Am J Med Sci 1942;204:625–48.
26. Coulam CB, Adamson SC, Annegers JF. Incidence of premature ovarian failure. Obstet Gynecol 1986;67(4):604–6.
27. Rebar RW, Connolly HV. Clinical features of young women with hypergonadotropic amenorrhea. Fertil Steril 1990;53(5):804–10.
28. Nelson LM, Anasti JN, Flack MR. Premature ovarian failure. Philadelphia: Lippincott–Raven; 1996.
29. Nelson LM, Kimzey LM, White BJ, et al. Gonadotropin suppression for the treatment of karyotypically normal spontaneous premature ovarian failure: a controlled trial. Fertil Steril 1992;57(1):50–5.
30. Aittomaki K, Lucena JL, Pakarinen P, et al. Mutation in the follicle-stimulating hormone receptor gene causes hereditary hypergonadotropic ovarian failure. Cell 1995;82(6):959–68.
31. Wolfsdorf JI, Rosenfield RL, Fang VS, et al. Partial gonadotrophin-resistance in pseudohypoparathyroidism. Acta Endocrinol (Copenh) 1978;88(2):321–8.
32. Yanase T, Simpson ER, Waterman MR. 17 alpha-hydroxylase/17,20-lyase deficiency: from clinical investigation to molecular definition. Endocr Rev 1991;12(1):91–108.
33. Hoek A, Schoemaker J, Drexhage HA. Premature ovarian failure and ovarian autoimmunity. Endocr Rev 1997;18(1):107–34.

34. Nelson LM, Anasti JN, Kimzey LM, et al. Development of luteinized graafian follicles in patients with karyotypically normal spontaneous premature ovarian failure. J Clin Endocrinol Metab 1994;79(5):1470–5.

35. Sybert VP, McCauley E. Turner's syndrome. N Engl J Med 2004;351(12): 1227–38.

36. Koh JM, Kim CH, Hong SK, et al. Primary ovarian failure caused by a solvent containing 2-bromopropane. Eur J Endocrinol 1998;138(5):554–6.

37. Di Pasquale E, Beck-Peccoz P, Persani L. Hypergonadotropic ovarian failure associated with an inherited mutation of human bone morphogenetic protein-15 (BMP15) gene. Am J Hum Genet 2004;75(1):106–11.

38. Bione S, Sala C, Manzini C, et al. A human homologue of the *Drosophila melanogaster* diaphanous gene is disrupted in a patient with premature ovarian failure: evidence for conserved function in oogenesis and implications for human sterility. Am J Hum Genet 1998;62(3):533–41.

39. Chand AL, Ooi GT, Harrison CA, et al. Functional analysis of the human inhibin alpha subunit variant A257T and its potential role in premature ovarian failure. Hum Reprod 2007;22(12):3241–8.

40. Toniolo D, Rizzolio F. X chromosome and ovarian failure. Semin Reprod Med 2007;25(4):264–71.

41. Smith JA, Vitale S, Reed GF, et al. Dry eye signs and symptoms in women with premature ovarian failure. Arch Ophthalmol 2004;122(2):151–6.

42. van Kasteren YM, Hundscheid RD, Smits AP, et al. Familial idiopathic premature ovarian failure: an overrated and underestimated genetic disease? Hum Reprod 1999;14(10):2455–9.

43. Wittenberger MD, Hagerman RJ, Sherman SL, et al. The FMR1 premutation and reproduction. Fertil Steril 2007;87(3):456–65.

44. Current evaluation of amenorrhea. Fertil Steril 2004;82(Suppl 1):S33–9.

45. Bakalov VK, Anasti JN, Calis KA, et al. Autoimmune oophoritis as a mechanism of follicular dysfunction in women with 46, XX spontaneous premature ovarian failure. Fertil Steril 2005;84(4):958–65.

46. Novosad JA, Kalantaridou SN, Tong ZB, et al. Ovarian antibodies as detected by indirect immunofluorescence are unreliable in the diagnosis of autoimmune premature ovarian failure: a controlled evaluation. BMC Womens Health 2003;3(1):2.

47. Rebar RW, Erickson GF, Yen SS. Idiopathic premature ovarian failure: clinical and endocrine characteristics. Fertil Steril 1982;37(1):35–41.

48. Greil AL. Infertility and psychological distress: a critical review of the literature. Soc Sci Med 1997;45(11):1679–704.

49. Kjaer TK, Jensen A, Dalton SO, et al. Suicide in Danish women evaluated for fertility problems. Hum Reprod 2011;26(9):2401–7.

50. Nelson LM. One world, one woman: a transformational leader's approach to primary ovarian insufficiency. Menopause 2011;18(5):480–7.

51. Davis M, Ventura JL, Wieners M, et al. The psychosocial transition associated with spontaneous 46, XX primary ovarian insufficiency: illness uncertainty, stigma, goal flexibility, and purpose in life as factors in emotional health. Fertil Steril 2010;93(7):2321–9.

52. Shuster LT, Rhodes DJ, Gostout BS, et al. Premature menopause or early menopause: long-term health consequences. Maturitas 2010;65(2):161–6.

53. Boughton MA. Premature menopause: multiple disruptions between the woman's biological body experience and her lived body. J Adv Nurs 2002;37(5):423–30.

54. Liao KL, Wood N, Conway GS. Premature menopause and psychological well-being. J Psychosom Obstet Gynaecol 2000;21(3):167–74.

55. Wright J, Allard M, Lecours A, et al. Psychosocial distress and infertility: a review of controlled research. Int J Fertil 1989;34(2):126–42.

56. Schmidt PJ, Cardoso GM, Ross JL, et al. Shyness, social anxiety, and impaired self-esteem in Turner syndrome and premature ovarian failure. JAMA 2006; 295(12):1374–6.

57. Orshan SA, Furniss KK, Forst C, et al. The lived experience of premature ovarian failure. J Obstet Gynecol Neonatal Nurs 2001;30(2):202–8.

58. Clayton PJ. Mortality and morbidity in the first year of widowhood. Arch Gen Psychiatry 1974;30(6):747–50.

59. Raphael B. The management of pathological grief. Aust N Z J Psychiatry 1975; 9(3):173–80.

60. Jacobs S, Hansen F, Kasl S, et al. Anxiety disorders during acute bereavement: risk and risk factors. J Clin Psychiatry 1990;51(7):269–74.

61. Downey G, Silver RC, Wortman CB. Reconsidering the attribution-adjustment relation following a major negative event: coping with the loss of a child. J Pers Soc Psychol 1990;59(5):925–40.

62. Horowitz MJ. A model of mourning: change in schemas of self and other. J Am Psychoanal Assoc 1990;38(2):297–324.

63. Stroebe M, Stroebe W. Does "grief work" work? J Consult Clin Psychol 1991; 59(3):479–82.

64. Prigerson HG, Frank E, Kasl SV, et al. Complicated grief and bereavement-related depression as distinct disorders: preliminary empirical validation in elderly bereaved spouses. Am J Psychiatry 1995;152(1):22–30.

65. Schmidt PJ, Luff JA, Haq NA, et al. Depression in women with spontaneous 46, XX primary ovarian insufficiency. J Clin Endocrinol Metab 2011;96(2):E278–87.

66. Orshan SA, Ventura JL, Covington SN, et al. Women with spontaneous 46, XX primary ovarian insufficiency (hypergonadotropic hypogonadism) have lower perceived social support than control women. Fertil Steril 2009;92(2):688–93.

67. Covington SN, Hillard PJ, Sterling EW, et al. A family systems approach to primary ovarian insufficiency. J Pediatr Adolesc Gynecol 2011;24(3):137–41.

68. Maslow A. Motivation and personality. 2nd edition. New York: Harper & Row; 1970.

69. Keyes CL, Shmotkin D, Ryff CD. Optimizing well-being: the empirical encounter of two traditions. J Pers Soc Psychol 2002;82(6):1007–22.

70. McGregor I, Little BR. Personal projects, happiness, and meaning: on doing well and being yourself. J Pers Soc Psychol 1998;74(2):494–512.

71. Frankl VE. From death-camp to existentialism a psychiatrist's path to a new therapy. Boston: Beacon Press; 1959.

72. Domar A, Penzias A, Dusek J, et al. The stress and distress of infertility: does religion help women cope? Sex Reprod Menopause 2005;3:45–51.

73. Ventura JL, Fitzgerald OR, Koziol DE, et al. Functional well-being is positively correlated with spiritual well-being in women who have spontaneous premature ovarian failure. Fertil Steril 2007;87(3):584–90.

74. Gallagher JC. Effect of early menopause on bone mineral density and fractures. Menopause 2007;14(3 Pt 2):567–71.

75. Jacobsen BK, Knutsen SF, Fraser GE. Age at natural menopause and total mortality and mortality from ischemic heart disease: the Adventist Health Study. J Clin Epidemiol 1999;52(4):303–7.

76. de Kleijn MJ, van der Schouw YT, Verbeek AL, et al. Endogenous estrogen exposure and cardiovascular mortality risk in postmenopausal women. Am J Epidemiol 2002;155(4):339–45.

77. Mondul AM, Rodriguez C, Jacobs EJ, et al. Age at natural menopause and cause-specific mortality. Am J Epidemiol 2005;162(11):1089–97.
78. Rossouw JE, Anderson GL, Prentice RL, et al. Risks and benefits of estrogen plus progestin in healthy postmenopausal women: principal results From the Women's Health Initiative randomized controlled trial. JAMA 2002;288(3):321–33.
79. Mishell DR Jr, Nakamura RM, Crosignani PG, et al. Serum gonadotropin and steroid patterns during the normal menstrual cycle. Am J Obstet Gynecol 1971;111(1):60–5.
80. Scarabin PY, Alhenc-Gelas M, Plu-Bureau G, et al. Effects of oral and transdermal estrogen/progesterone regimens on blood coagulation and fibrinolysis in postmenopausal women. A randomized controlled trial. Arterioscler Thromb Vasc Biol 1997;17(11):3071–8.
81. Scarabin PY, Oger E, Plu-Bureau G. Differential association of oral and transdermal oestrogen-replacement therapy with venous thromboembolism risk. Lancet 2003;362(9382):428–32.
82. Canonico M, Oger E, Plu-Bureau G, et al. Hormone therapy and venous thromboembolism among postmenopausal women: impact of the route of estrogen administration and progestogens: the ESTHER study. Circulation 2007;115(7): 840–5.
83. Gibbons WE, Moyer DL, Lobo RA, et al. Biochemical and histologic effects of sequential estrogen/progestin therapy on the endometrium of postmenopausal women. Am J Obstet Gynecol 1986;154(2):456–61.
84. Bjarnason K, Cerin A, Lindgren R, et al. Adverse endometrial effects during long cycle hormone replacement therapy. Scandinavian Long Cycle Study Group. Maturitas 1999;32(3):161–70.
85. van Kasteren YM, Schoemaker J. Premature ovarian failure: a systematic review on therapeutic interventions to restore ovarian function and achieve pregnancy. Hum Reprod Update 1999;5(5):483–92.
86. Pines A, Sturdee DW, Birkhauser MH, et al. IMS updated recommendations on postmenopausal hormone therapy. Climacteric 2007;10(3):181–94.
87. McConkie-Rosell A, Finucane B, Cronister A, et al. Genetic counseling for fragile x syndrome: updated recommendations of the national society of genetic counselors. J Genet Couns 2005;14(4):249–70.
88. Sherman S, Pletcher BA, Driscoll DA. Fragile X syndrome: diagnostic and carrier testing. Genet Med 2005;7(8):584–7.
89. American College of Obstetricians and Gynecologists Committee on Genetics. ACOG Committee Opinion. No. 338. Screening for fragile X syndrome. Obstet Gynecol 2006;107(6):1483–5.
90. Popat VB, Calis KA, Vanderhoof VH, et al. Bone mineral density in estrogen-deficient young women. J Clin Endocrinol Metab 2009;94(7):2277–83.
91. North American Menopause Society. The role of calcium in peri- and postmenopausal women: 2006 position statement of the North American Menopause Society. Menopause 2006;13(6):862–77 [quiz: 878–80].
92. Martyn-St James M, Carroll S. A meta-analysis of impact exercise on postmenopausal bone loss: the case for mixed loading exercise programmes. Br J Sports Med 2009;43(12):898–908.
93. Holick MF. Vitamin D deficiency. N Engl J Med 2007;357(3):266–81.
94. Drake MT, Clarke BL, Khosla S. Bisphosphonates: mechanism of action and role in clinical practice. Mayo Clin Proc 2008;83(9):1032–45.
95. Floyd RL, O'Connor MJ, Sokol RJ, et al. Recognition and prevention of fetal alcohol syndrome. Obstet Gynecol 2005;106(5 Pt 1):1059–64.

96. ACOG Committee on Ethics. ACOG Committee Opinion. Number 294, May 2004. At-risk drinking and illicit drug use: ethical issues in obstetric and gynecologic practice. Obstet Gynecol 2004;103(5 Pt 1):1021–31.
97. ACOG Committee on Health Care for Underdeserved Women; ACOG Committee on Obstetric Practice. ACOG Committee Opinion. Number 316, October 2005. Smoking cessation during pregnancy. Obstet Gynecol 2005;106(4):883–8.
98. The American Academy of Pediatrics and The American College of Obstetricians and Gynecologists. Guidelines for Perinatal Care. 5th edition. Elk Grove Village (IL): American Academy of Pediatrics; 2002.
99. Stazi AV, Mantovani A. A risk factor for female fertility and pregnancy: celiac disease. Gynecol Endocrinol 2000;14(6):454–63.
100. Bakalov VK, Vanderhoof VH, Bondy CA, et al. Adrenal antibodies detect asymptomatic auto-immune adrenal insufficiency in young women with spontaneous premature ovarian failure. Hum Reprod 2002;17(8):2096–100.
101. Kim TJ, Anasti JN, Flack MR, et al. Routine endocrine screening for patients with karyotypically normal spontaneous premature ovarian failure. Obstet Gynecol 1997;89(5 Pt 1):777–9.
102. Baker V. Life plans and family-building options for women with primary ovarian insufficiency. Semin Reprod Med 2011;29(4):362–72.
103. Miall C. The stigma of involuntary childlessness. Soc Probl 1986;33:268–82.
104. Whiteford LM, Gonzalez L. Stigma: the hidden burden of infertility. Soc Sci Med 1995;40(1):27–36.
105. Lovett LL. Conceiving the future: pronatalism, reproduction, and the family in the United States, 1890-1938. Chapel Hill (NC): University of North Carolina Press; 2007.
106. Greil AL, Porter KL, Leitko TL, et al. Why me?: theodicies of infertile women and men. Sociol Health Illn 1989;11:213–29.
107. Becker G. Metaphors in disrupted lives: Infertility and cultural constructions of continuity. Med Anthropol Q 1994;8:383–410.
108. Woollett A. Childlessness: strategies for coping with infertility. Int J Behav Dev 1985;8:473–82.
109. Alper MM, Jolly EE, Garner PR. Pregnancies after premature ovarian failure. Obstet Gynecol 1986;67(Suppl 3):59S–62S.
110. Hafez ES, Evans TN. Human reproduction, conception and contraception. Hagerstown (MD): Medical Dept: Harper & Row; 1973.
111. Silber SJ, Grudzinskas G, Gosden RG. Successful pregnancy after microsurgical transplantation of an intact ovary. N Engl J Med 2008;359(24):2617–8.
112. Sauer MV, Paulson RJ, Lobo RA. A preliminary report on oocyte donation extending reproductive potential to women over 40. N Engl J Med 1990;323(17):1157–60.
113. Soderstrom-Anttila V, Tiitinen A, Foudila T, et al. Obstetric and perinatal outcome after oocyte donation: comparison with in-vitro fertilization pregnancies. Hum Reprod 1998;13(2):483–90.
114. Salha O, Sharma V, Dada T, et al. The influence of donated gametes on the incidence of hypertensive disorders of pregnancy. Hum Reprod 1999;14(9):2268–73.
115. Krieg SA, Henne MB, Westphal LM. Obstetric outcomes in donor oocyte pregnancies compared with advanced maternal age in in vitro fertilization pregnancies. Fertil Steril 2008;90(1):65–70.
116. Keenan J, Finger R, Check JH, et al. Favorable pregnancy, delivery, and implantation rates experienced in embryo donation programs in the United States. Fertil Steril 2008;90(4):1077–80.

117. Hartigan EG, Brown DJ. Discharge planning for continuity of care. The service population. NLN Publ 1985;(20–1977):19–27.
118. Mc carthy S. Discharge planning: strategies for assuring continuity of care. Rockville (MD): Aspen; 1988.
119. Moore M, Ekman E, Shumway M. Understanding the critical role of social work in safety net medical settings: framework for research and practice in the emergency department. Soc Work Health Care 2012;51(2):140–8.
120. Galati M, Wong HJ, Morra D, et al. An evidence-based case for the value of social workers in efficient hospital discharge. Health Care Manag (Frederick) 2011;30(3):242–6.

Index

Note: Page numbers of article titles are in **boldface** type.

Obstet Gynecol Clin N Am 39 (2012) 587–594
http://dx.doi.org/10.1016/S0889-8545(12)00094-0
0889-8545/12/$ – see front matter © 2012 Elsevier Inc. All rights reserved.

obgyn.theclinics.com

United States Postal Service

Statement of Ownership, Management, and Circulation
(All Periodicals Publications Except Requestor Publications)

1. Publication Title
Obstetrics and Gynecology Clinics of North America

2. Publication Number
0 0 0 - 2 7 6

3. Filing Date
9/14/12

4. Issue Frequency
Mar, Jun, Sep, Dec

5. Number of Issues Published Annually
4

6. Annual Subscription Price
$293.00

7. Complete Mailing Address of Known Office of Publication (Not printer) (Street, city, county, state, and ZIP+4®)

Elsevier Inc.
360 Park Avenue South
New York, NY 10010-1710

Contact Person
Stephen R. Bushing

Telephone (Include area code)
215-239-3688

8. Complete Mailing Address of Headquarters or General Business Office of Publisher (Not printer)

Elsevier Inc., 360 Park Avenue South, New York, NY 10010-1710

9. Full Names and Complete Mailing Addresses of Publisher, Editor, and Managing Editor (Do not leave blank)

Publisher (Name and complete mailing address)
Kim Murphy, Elsevier, Inc., 1600 John F. Kennedy Blvd. Suite 1800, Philadelphia, PA 19103-2899

Editor (Name and complete mailing address)
Stephanie Donley, Elsevier, Inc., 1600 John F. Kennedy Blvd. Suite 1800, Philadelphia, PA 19103-2899

Managing Editor (Name and complete mailing address)
Sarah Barth, Elsevier, Inc., 1600 John F. Kennedy Blvd. Suite 1800, Philadelphia, PA 19103-2899

10. Owner (Do not leave blank. If the publication is owned by a corporation, give the name and address of the corporation immediately followed by the names and addresses of all stockholders owning or holding 1 percent or more of the total amount of stock. If not owned by a corporation, give the names and addresses of the individual owners. If owned by a partnership or other unincorporated firm, give its name and address as well as those of each individual owner. If the publication is published by a nonprofit organization, give its name and address.)

Full Name	Complete Mailing Address
Wholly owned subsidiary of	1600 John F. Kennedy Blvd., Ste. 1800
Reed/Elsevier, US holdings	Philadelphia, PA 19103-2899

11. Known Bondholders, Mortgagees, and Other Security Holders Owning or Holding 1 Percent or More of Total Amount of Bonds, Mortgages, or Other Securities. If none, check box ☑ None

Full Name	Complete Mailing Address
N/A	

12. Tax Status (For completion by nonprofit organizations authorized to mail at nonprofit rates) (Check one)
The purpose, function, and nonprofit status of this organization and the exempt status for federal income tax purposes:
☐ Has Not Changed During Preceding 12 Months
☐ Has Changed During Preceding 12 Months (Publisher must submit explanation of change with this statement)

PS Form 3526, September 2007 (Page 1 of 3 (Instructions Page 3)) PSN 7530-01-000-9931 PRIVACY NOTICE: See our Privacy policy in www.usps.com

---

13. Publication Title
Obstetrics and Gynecology Clinics of North America

14. Issue Date for Circulation Data Below
September 2012

15. Extent and Nature of Circulation

			Average No. Copies Each Issue During Preceding 12 Months	No. Copies of Single Issue Published Nearest to Filing Date
a. Total Number of Copies (Net press run)			1013	904
b. Paid Circulation (By Mail and Outside the Mail)	(1)	Mailed Outside-County Paid Subscriptions Stated on PS Form 3541. (Include paid distribution above nominal rate, advertiser's proof copies, and exchange copies)	302	273
	(2)	Mailed In-County Paid Subscriptions Stated on PS Form 3541 (Include paid distribution above nominal rate, advertiser's proof copies, and exchange copies)		
	(3)	Paid Distribution Outside the Mails Including Sales Through Dealers and Carriers, Street Vendors, Counter Sales, and Other Paid Distribution Outside USPS®	320	350
	(4)	Paid Distribution by Other Classes Mailed Through the USPS (e.g. First-Class Mail®)		
c. Total Paid Distribution (Sum of 15b (1), (2), (3), and (4))		▶	622	623
d. Free or Nominal Rate Distribution (By Mail and Outside the Mail)	(1)	Free or Nominal Rate Outside-County Copies Included on PS Form 3541	77	66
	(2)	Free or Nominal Rate In-County Copies Included on PS Form 3541		
	(3)	Free or Nominal Rate Copies Mailed at Other Classes Through the USPS (e.g. First-Class Mail)		
	(4)	Free or Nominal Rate Distribution Outside the Mail (Carriers or other means)		
e. Total Free or Nominal Rate Distribution (Sum of 15d (1), (2), (3) and (4))		▶	77	66
f. Total Distribution (Sum of 15c and 15e)		▶	699	689
g. Copies not Distributed (See instructions to publishers #4 (page #3))		▶	314	215
h. Total (Sum of 15f and g)		▶	1013	904
i. Percent Paid (15c divided by 15f times 100)		▶	88.98%	90.42%

16. Publication of Statement of Ownership
☐ If the publication is a general publication, publication of this statement is required. Will be printed in the December 2012 issue of this publication. ☐ Publication not required.

17. Signature and Title of Editor, Publisher, Business Manager, or Owner

[signature] Stephen R. Bushing - Inventory/Distribution Coordinator

Date September 14, 2012

I certify that all information furnished on this form is true and complete. I understand that anyone who furnishes false or misleading information on this form or who omits material or information requested on the form may be subject to criminal sanctions (including fines and imprisonment) and/or civil sanctions (including civil penalties).

PS Form 3526, September 2007 (Page 2 of 3)

Moving?

Make sure your subscription moves with you!

To notify us of your new address, find your **Clinics Account Number** (located on your mailing label above your name), and contact customer service at:

Email: journalscustomerservice-usa@elsevier.com

800-654-2452 (subscribers in the U.S. & Canada)
314-447-8871 (subscribers outside of the U.S. & Canada)

Fax number: 314-447-8029

Elsevier Health Sciences Division
Subscription Customer Service
3251 Riverport Lane
Maryland Heights, MO 63043

ELSEVIER

Printed and bound by CPI Group (UK) Ltd, Croydon, CR0 4YY

03/10/2024

01040460-0010